PTCB EXAM STUDY GUIDE

Master the Pharmacy Technician Certification Exam with Expert Tips & Strategies, 200+ Flashcards, and 5 Full-Length Practice Tests with Over 400 Q&A for Effortless Success

Harrison Academic Press

TABLE OF CONTENTS

1. INTRODUCTION

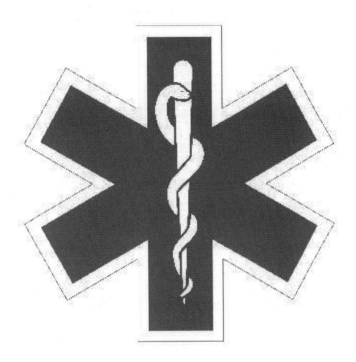

HOW TO MAXIMIZE YOUR USE OF THIS GUIDE

Embarking on your journey to become a certified pharmacy technician is both an exciting and challenging endeavor. This guide is your trusted companion, meticulously designed to help you navigate the complexities of the PTCB exam and emerge victorious. To make the most of this resource, it's essential to understand how to effectively utilize each section, implement the strategies provided, and tailor the content to fit your unique learning style and schedule.

First and foremost, approach this guide as your personalized roadmap. Think of it as a mentor guiding you through the labyrinth of pharmacy knowledge, ready to provide insights and encouragement at every turn. The structure of this guide is intentionally crafted to build your understanding progressively, starting with foundational concepts and moving towards more complex topics. This logical flow ensures that you establish a solid base before tackling advanced material, preventing overwhelm and fostering confidence.

Begin by familiarizing yourself with the Table of Contents. This comprehensive outline is not just a list of chapters; it's your strategic plan. Each chapter is designed to cover specific areas of the PTCB exam, from the essentials of pharmacology to the nuances of pharmacy operations and financial management. By understanding the layout, you can prioritize sections based on your strengths and weaknesses, dedicating more time to areas where you need additional practice.

One of the key strategies for maximizing your use of this guide is to integrate active learning techniques. Passive reading is rarely sufficient for retaining complex information. Instead, engage with the material dynamically. As you read through each chapter, take notes, highlight key concepts, and summarize sections in your own words. These actions reinforce learning and help transfer information from short-term to long-term memory.

Incorporate the practice questions and flashcards provided at the end of chapters and within the supplementary materials. These tools are not mere add-ons; they are integral to your study regimen. Practice questions mimic the format and style of the PTCB exam, offering you a realistic preview of what to expect. Use them to test your knowledge regularly, identify gaps, and gauge your progress. Flashcards are particularly effective for memorizing drug names, classifications, and pharmacy laws, enabling quick recall during the exam.

Equally important is the establishment of a consistent study schedule. Consistency is the bedrock of effective learning. Craft a study plan that aligns with your daily routine, ensuring regular, uninterrupted study periods. Whether you're an early bird or a night owl, find your most productive hours and dedicate them to studying. Break your study sessions into manageable chunks, focusing on one chapter or subchapter at a time. This approach prevents burnout and allows for deep, concentrated learning.

Remember to incorporate breaks and downtime into your schedule. The brain requires rest to process and consolidate information. Short, frequent breaks during study sessions can enhance focus and retention. Additionally, ensure you get adequate sleep, maintain a balanced diet, and engage in physical activity. A healthy body supports a sharp mind, crucial for mastering the extensive content required for the PTCB exam.

Another effective strategy is to apply the knowledge gained in real-world scenarios. If you're currently working in a pharmacy setting, try to connect what you learn with your daily tasks. This contextual learning solidifies concepts and makes them more relatable and easier to recall. Discussing topics with colleagues or joining study groups can also provide different perspectives and deepen your understanding.

Throughout your preparation, it's essential to stay motivated and optimistic. The journey to certification can be long and, at times, arduous. Set clear, attainable goals and reward yourself for reaching milestones. Celebrate small victories, whether it's mastering a challenging concept or achieving a high score on a practice test. Maintaining a positive mindset will keep you energized and resilient, even when faced with difficult topics.

This guide also emphasizes the importance of mental and physical preparation. Exam day can be stressful, but proper preparation can mitigate anxiety. Familiarize yourself with the exam format, understand the types of questions you'll encounter, and develop strategies for managing your time during the test. Visualization techniques and mindfulness exercises can help calm nerves and enhance concentration.

It's also crucial to keep in mind that learning is an iterative process. Don't be discouraged by mistakes or setbacks. Each error is an opportunity to learn and improve. Review incorrect answers on practice tests to understand where you went wrong and revisit those topics in the guide. This process of continual improvement will gradually build your competence and confidence.

Lastly, leverage the additional resources and support provided within this guide. References to authoritative texts, online resources, and professional organizations offer avenues for further exploration. Joining forums or online communities for pharmacy technicians can provide additional support, insights, and motivation from peers who are on the same journey.

In conclusion, maximizing your use of this guide involves a strategic, active, and holistic approach to learning. Embrace this guide as your ally, engage deeply with the content, and remain consistent and positive in your study efforts. By doing so, you will not only be well-prepared to pass the PTCB exam but also equipped with the knowledge and skills to excel in your pharmacy technician career. Your journey to certification is a significant step towards a rewarding and impactful profession, and this guide is here to ensure you reach that destination with confidence and success.

COMPREHENSIVE OVERVIEW OF THE PTCB EXAM

The Pharmacy Technician Certification Board (PTCB) exam is a pivotal milestone for anyone aspiring to become a certified pharmacy technician. Understanding the comprehensive landscape of this exam is crucial for your preparation and success. This overview will provide you with a clear picture of what to expect, demystifying the process and setting you on a confident path towards certification.

The PTCB exam, formally known as the Pharmacy Technician Certification Exam (PTCE), is designed to evaluate the knowledge and skills necessary for a pharmacy technician to effectively assist pharmacists in their daily tasks. It ensures that candidates possess the essential competencies required to perform their duties safely and efficiently. Passing this exam not only validates your expertise but also opens doors to better job opportunities and career advancement.

At its core, the PTCE assesses your proficiency across several domains of pharmacy practice. These domains include medications, federal requirements, patient safety and quality assurance, and order entry and processing. Each domain is crucial, reflecting the diverse responsibilities you will encounter in a pharmacy setting. Let's delve into each of these domains to give you a comprehensive understanding of the exam's structure and content.

The first domain, Medications, encompasses about 40% of the exam. This section tests your knowledge of drug names, both generic and brand, their uses, dosages, side effects, and interactions. Understanding medications is fundamental to your role as a pharmacy technician. You'll need to be familiar with the various classes of drugs, their mechanisms of action, and the therapeutic outcomes they are intended to achieve. This knowledge ensures you can accurately assist in dispensing medications and provide appropriate information to patients.

Federal Requirements constitute approximately 12.5% of the exam. This domain covers the laws and regulations that govern pharmacy practice in the United States. You'll need to be well-versed in the Controlled Substances Act, the Food, Drug, and Cosmetic Act, and other relevant federal legislation. This knowledge is critical for maintaining compliance with legal standards and ensuring the safe handling of medications. Understanding these requirements helps prevent errors and safeguards patient health.

Patient Safety and Quality Assurance is another significant domain, making up about 26.25% of the exam. This section focuses on practices that ensure the safety and well-being of patients. It includes topics such as error prevention strategies, medication storage and handling, and quality control procedures. Patient safety is paramount in pharmacy practice, and this domain tests your ability to implement protocols that minimize risks and enhance the quality of care provided.

Order Entry and Processing, accounting for 21.25% of the exam, evaluates your competency in the technical aspects of pharmacy operations. This includes interpreting prescriptions, inputting orders into the pharmacy information system, and ensuring the accuracy of medication dispensing. Proficiency in this domain is essential for maintaining an efficient workflow and preventing errors that could adversely affect patient outcomes.

The PTCE consists of 90 multiple-choice questions, with 80 scored and 10 unscored questions. The unscored questions are included to gather statistical data for future exams and do not affect your final score. The exam is computer-based and administered at Pearson VUE test centers nationwide. You will have two hours to complete the exam, which includes a short tutorial and post-exam survey.

Understanding the format and content of the PTCE is just the beginning. Effective preparation requires a strategic approach. Start by assessing your strengths and weaknesses in each domain. This self-evaluation will help you prioritize your study efforts, dedicating more time to areas where you need improvement. Use the practice questions and flashcards included in this guide to reinforce your knowledge and identify areas that require further review.

Developing a solid study plan is also crucial. Allocate specific times for studying each domain, ensuring a balanced approach that covers all content areas. Consistency is key, so establish a regular study routine that fits your schedule. Incorporate active learning techniques such as summarizing information in your own words, teaching concepts to a friend or family member, and applying knowledge to real-world scenarios.

In addition to studying the content, it's important to familiarize yourself with the exam's logistics. Registering for the PTCE involves a few straightforward steps. First, create an account on the PTCB website and complete the application process. Ensure you meet the eligibility requirements, which include a high school diploma or equivalent and full disclosure of all criminal and State Board of Pharmacy registration or licensure actions. Once your application is approved, you can schedule your exam at a Pearson VUE test center.

On exam day, arrive at the test center early to allow time for check-in procedures. Bring two forms of valid identification, one of which must be a government-issued photo ID. Personal belongings, including electronic devices and study materials, are not permitted in the testing area, so plan accordingly. The test center will provide you with a locker to store your belongings.

During the exam, manage your time effectively. With 90 questions to answer in 120 minutes, you have an average of 1.3 minutes per question. Pace yourself to ensure you have enough time to review your answers. Read each question carefully, and use the process of elimination to narrow down your choices. If you encounter a difficult question, make your best guess and move on. You can flag questions to revisit if time permits.

After completing the exam, you'll receive an unofficial score report indicating whether you passed or failed. The official score report will be available on your PTCB account within a few weeks. If you pass, congratulations! You'll receive your certification and can begin using the CPhT (Certified Pharmacy Technician) credential. If you do not pass, don't be discouraged. Use the experience as a learning opportunity, review your performance, and focus on improving in weaker areas before retaking the exam.

In conclusion, the PTCB exam is a comprehensive assessment that evaluates your knowledge and skills across critical domains of pharmacy practice. Understanding the structure and content of the exam is essential for effective preparation. By strategically studying each domain, familiarizing yourself with the exam format, and managing your time efficiently, you can approach the PTCE with confidence. Remember, this guide is your ally in this journey, providing you with the knowledge, tools, and support needed to succeed. With dedication and perseverance, you'll be well-equipped to pass the exam and take a significant step forward in your pharmacy technician career.

MENTAL AND PHYSICAL PREPARATION STRATEGIES

As you prepare to tackle the Pharmacy Technician Certification Exam (PTCE), it's essential to focus not only on your intellectual readiness but also on your mental and physical well-being. Successfully navigating the exam requires a holistic approach that balances rigorous study with effective stress management and self-care. This chapter will guide you through strategies to ensure you're mentally sharp and physically resilient on exam day.

The journey to becoming a certified pharmacy technician begins with a commitment to your mental health. The pressure of studying for a high-stakes exam can be overwhelming, but with the right mindset, you can transform anxiety into motivation. Start by setting realistic goals. Break down your study plan into manageable chunks, celebrating small victories along the way. This approach prevents burnout and keeps you motivated. Remember, it's not about cramming all the information at once but building your knowledge steadily over time.

Creating a positive study environment is crucial for maintaining focus and reducing stress. Choose a quiet, well-lit space free from distractions. Equip your study area with all necessary materials—books, notes, flashcards, and practice tests. The act of organizing your space can itself be a calming ritual, signaling to your brain that it's time to focus. Consistency is key; try to study at the same time each day to establish a routine that becomes second nature.

Incorporate mindfulness techniques into your daily routine. Mindfulness is about being present in the moment, fully engaged with whatever you're doing. Simple practices like deep breathing, meditation, or even mindful walking can significantly reduce anxiety and improve concentration. Start your study sessions with a few minutes of mindfulness to clear your mind and set a calm, focused tone for your work.

Another powerful mental preparation strategy is visualization. Spend a few minutes each day visualizing yourself successfully completing the exam. Imagine the testing environment, the process of answering questions confidently, and the relief and joy of seeing your passing score. Visualization can program your mind for success, building confidence and reducing fear of the unknown.

Your physical health is just as important as your mental state. Regular physical activity boosts brain function, improves mood, and helps manage stress. You don't need to engage in strenuous exercise; even a daily walk, yoga session, or short workout can have significant benefits. Find an activity you enjoy and make it a regular part of your routine. Exercise not only keeps your body fit but also increases blood flow to the brain, enhancing cognitive function and memory.

Nutrition plays a critical role in your ability to study effectively and perform well on exam day. Aim for a balanced diet rich in fruits, vegetables, lean proteins, and whole grains. These foods provide the necessary nutrients for optimal brain function. Stay hydrated by drinking plenty of water throughout the day. Avoid excessive caffeine and sugar, which can lead to energy crashes and impair concentration.

Sleep is another cornerstone of physical preparation. During sleep, your brain processes and consolidates information, making it easier to recall what you've learned. Aim for seven to nine hours of quality sleep each night. Establish a regular sleep schedule, going to bed and waking up at the same time each day. Create a relaxing bedtime routine to signal to your body that it's time to wind down. Avoid screens and stimulating activities before bed, as they can interfere with your ability to fall asleep.

As exam day approaches, it's normal to feel a mix of excitement and anxiety. Managing this emotional rollercoaster is essential for maintaining focus and performing your best. One effective strategy is to develop a pre-exam routine that calms your nerves and prepares your mind. This routine might include a light review of materials, a healthy breakfast, some gentle exercise, and a few minutes of mindfulness or visualization. Sticking to a routine can provide a sense of normalcy and control amidst the high stakes of exam day.

On the day before the exam, prioritize relaxation and rest over last-minute cramming. Trust in the preparation you've done. Engage in activities that you find calming and enjoyable—whether that's reading a book, watching a favorite movie, or spending time with loved ones. Make sure to get a good night's sleep so you wake up refreshed and ready to tackle the exam.

When exam day arrives, begin with a balanced breakfast that provides sustained energy. Complex carbohydrates like oatmeal or whole-grain toast, combined with protein such as eggs or yogurt, can keep you full and focused. Arrive at the testing center early to allow time for check-in procedures and to settle in without feeling rushed.

During the exam, remember to pace yourself. It's easy to get caught up in the pressure and rush through questions, but this can lead to careless mistakes. Read each question carefully and take your time to consider all options before answering. If you encounter a particularly challenging question, don't panic. Mark it and move on, returning to it after you've answered the easier questions. This strategy ensures you maximize your time and maintain momentum.

In moments of stress or self-doubt during the exam, use deep breathing techniques to calm your mind. Take a few slow, deep breaths, focusing on the sensation of the air filling your lungs and then slowly exhaling. This simple practice can help clear your mind, reduce anxiety, and refocus your attention.

Post-exam, it's important to practice self-compassion, regardless of the outcome. Reflect on your effort and dedication throughout the preparation process. Acknowledge your hard work and resilience. If the results aren't what you hoped for, don't be disheartened. Analyze your performance, identify areas for improvement, and create a plan for moving forward. Remember, setbacks are part of the learning journey and can provide valuable lessons for future success.

In conclusion, mental and physical preparation for the PTCE is about more than just studying hard. It's about fostering a positive mindset, creating a conducive learning environment, maintaining a healthy lifestyle, and developing effective stress management techniques. By integrating these strategies into your routine, you can approach the exam with confidence, knowing you're fully prepared to succeed. Your journey to becoming a certified pharmacy technician is as much about personal growth as it is about professional achievement, and taking care of your mental and physical well-being is a critical part of that journey.

SETTING UP YOUR STUDY PLAN

Setting up an effective study plan is the cornerstone of your preparation for the Pharmacy Technician Certification Exam (PTCE). With a structured and personalized approach, you can navigate the vast amount of material with confidence and efficiency. A well-thought-out study plan will help you manage your time, stay organized, and ensure comprehensive coverage of all exam topics. Let's embark on this journey together, creating a roadmap that leads to your success.

Begin by understanding your current situation and availability. Assess your daily schedule and identify time slots that can be dedicated to studying. Consider your work hours, family commitments, and personal activities. It's important to be realistic about how much time you can commit each day. Whether you have two hours or just thirty minutes, consistency is key. Establishing a routine will help you build momentum and make studying a habitual part of your day.

Next, set clear, achievable goals for your study sessions. Break down the entire syllabus into smaller, manageable sections. For instance, allocate specific days for different domains of the exam such as medications, federal requirements, and patient safety. This approach prevents the material from becoming overwhelming and allows for focused, in-depth study of each topic. Setting daily or weekly goals can also provide a sense of accomplishment and keep you motivated as you progress.

To maintain a structured plan, create a study calendar. This visual representation of your schedule can be a powerful tool for organization. Mark important dates, such as the exam day, and work backwards to allocate time for each subject. Include milestones for completing practice tests and reviewing flashcards. A calendar not only keeps you on track but also serves as a motivational reminder of your commitment to this journey.

Variety is crucial in your study plan to keep your mind engaged and prevent burnout. Mix up your study methods by incorporating different resources and activities. For example, combine reading the textbook with watching instructional videos, participating in study groups, and using interactive online quizzes. Diversifying your approach caters to different learning styles and reinforces your understanding of the material.

Incorporate regular review sessions into your plan. Revisiting topics periodically helps reinforce knowledge and aids long-term retention. Use techniques like spaced repetition, which involves reviewing material at increasing intervals, to enhance memory. This method is particularly effective for mastering the vast array of drug names and classifications required for the PTCE.

Balance is also essential in your study plan. It's important to intersperse periods of intense focus with breaks. Studies have shown that short breaks during study sessions can improve concentration and productivity. The Pomodoro Technique, for example, involves studying for 25 minutes followed by a 5-minute break. After four cycles, take a longer break of 15-30 minutes. This technique helps maintain high levels of mental clarity and prevents fatigue.

While self-study is important, don't underestimate the value of collaborative learning. Joining a study group can provide different perspectives, clarify doubts, and keep you accountable. Discussing topics with peers can deepen your understanding and reveal areas you might have overlooked. Online forums and local study groups are great places to connect with fellow candidates preparing for the PTCE.

Flexibility is another critical component of an effective study plan. Life is unpredictable, and there may be days when sticking to your schedule is challenging. It's important to be adaptable and adjust your plan as needed. If you miss a study session, don't stress. Simply reorganize your schedule to make up for lost time. Flexibility ensures that unexpected events don't derail your overall progress.

Leverage the power of technology to enhance your study plan. There are numerous apps and tools designed to aid in exam preparation. Apps like Quizlet allow you to create and study flashcards on the go, while platforms like Khan Academy offer comprehensive tutorials on relevant subjects. Additionally, many websites provide practice tests that simulate the exam environment, helping you build familiarity and confidence.

As you approach the final weeks before the exam, intensify your preparation. Use this time for thorough revision, focusing on areas where you feel less confident. Take full-length practice exams under timed conditions to gauge your readiness and improve your time management skills. Analyzing your performance on these tests can highlight strengths and areas needing improvement, guiding your final review sessions.

Remember, your study plan should also account for self-care. Preparing for the PTCE is a marathon, not a sprint. Ensuring you get enough sleep, eat nutritious meals, and engage in regular physical activity is vital for maintaining your overall well-being. A healthy body supports a sharp mind, enhancing your ability to absorb and retain information.

Positive reinforcement plays a significant role in maintaining motivation. Celebrate your achievements, no matter how small. Reward yourself for reaching milestones and completing difficult sections. These rewards can be simple, like treating yourself to your favorite snack, taking a relaxing walk, or enjoying a leisure activity. Recognizing your progress keeps your spirits high and reinforces your commitment to the journey.

Additionally, seek support from friends, family, and mentors. Sharing your goals and progress with others can provide encouragement and accountability. They can offer valuable perspectives, help you stay motivated, and provide a support system during challenging times. Don't hesitate to ask for help or guidance when needed.

In summary, setting up a study plan for the PTCE involves a blend of strategic organization, diverse study methods, and a commitment to self-care. By assessing your schedule, setting clear goals, and incorporating various resources and techniques, you can create a robust plan that caters to your unique needs. Flexibility, regular reviews, and collaborative learning further enhance your preparation. Balancing study with personal well-being ensures you remain focused and energized throughout your journey. With a well-crafted study plan, you'll be well-equipped to tackle the PTCE confidently and achieve your goal of becoming a certified pharmacy technician.

2. EXAM ESSENTIALS

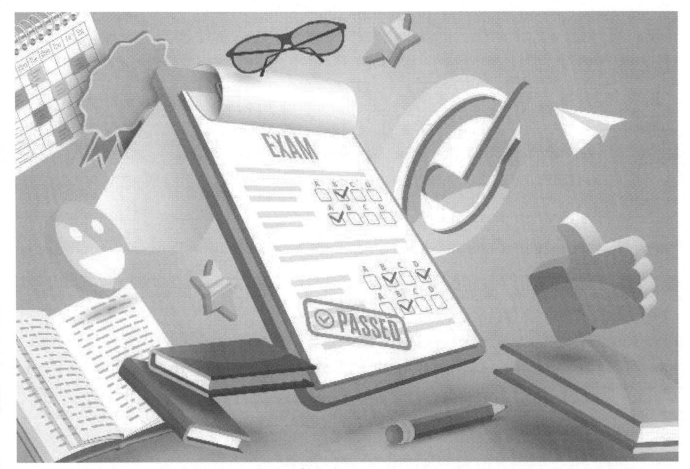

Understanding the essentials of the PTCB exam is a crucial step in your journey to becoming a certified pharmacy technician. This chapter is designed to demystify the process, guiding you through the key aspects of what you need to know before the big day. From who is eligible to take the exam, to the specifics of registration and the format of the test, we'll cover every detail to ensure you are fully prepared.

Imagine stepping into the exam room with confidence, knowing exactly what to expect. That sense of assurance comes from being well-informed and thoroughly prepared. We'll explore the eligibility criteria to confirm you meet all requirements, walk you through the registration process to eliminate any last-minute surprises, and provide a clear understanding of the exam format and content.

As you delve into this chapter, picture yourself navigating the exam process smoothly, from registration to test day. Visualize knowing how to manage your time effectively and approach each question with calm and clarity. With this comprehensive overview, you'll be equipped not only with the knowledge to succeed but also with the peace of mind that comes from thorough preparation. Let's take this step together, setting the foundation for your success on the PTCB exam.

WHO CAN TAKE THE PTCB EXAM?

The journey to becoming a certified pharmacy technician begins with understanding the eligibility criteria for the PTCB exam. Knowing whether you qualify to take the exam is the first step on this path, and it sets the stage for all the preparation that follows. Let's explore who can take the PTCB exam, ensuring you're fully informed and ready to proceed with confidence.

The Pharmacy Technician Certification Exam (PTCE) is designed for individuals who seek to demonstrate their knowledge and skills in pharmacy practice. To be eligible, candidates must meet specific criteria set forth by the Pharmacy Technician Certification Board (PTCB). These requirements ensure that all candidates possess a baseline level of education and experience necessary to perform effectively in a pharmacy setting.

First and foremost, candidates must have a high school diploma or equivalent. This requirement underscores the importance of foundational education in supporting the complex responsibilities of a pharmacy technician. The high school diploma ensures that candidates have achieved a general level of education and are equipped with basic skills in reading, writing, and mathematics—skills that are crucial for understanding and managing pharmaceutical tasks.

In addition to educational qualifications, the PTCB requires candidates to have completed a pharmacy technician training program or possess equivalent work experience. This requirement can be fulfilled in several ways. Many candidates complete formal training programs offered by community colleges, vocational schools, or online education providers. These programs typically cover essential topics such as pharmacology, pharmacy law, and medication management, providing a comprehensive foundation for aspiring pharmacy technicians.

For those who have gained experience through employment, equivalent work experience can also meet the eligibility criteria. If you've worked as a pharmacy technician under the supervision of a licensed pharmacist, your hands-on experience may qualify you to take the exam. This path recognizes the value of practical experience and on-the-job learning, acknowledging that skills developed in real-world settings are equally valid.

However, eligibility isn't just about educational background and work experience. The PTCB also emphasizes the importance of ethical behavior and professionalism. Candidates must disclose any criminal convictions or State Board of Pharmacy registration or licensure actions. This transparency is vital because pharmacy technicians hold positions of trust, handling sensitive information and medications. The PTCB aims to ensure that all certified technicians adhere to high ethical standards, safeguarding patient safety and maintaining public trust in the profession.

Once you've determined that you meet the educational and ethical criteria, the next step is to apply for the exam. The application process is straightforward but requires attention to detail. You'll need to create an account on the PTCB website and complete the application form, providing information about your educational background, training, and work experience. Be sure to gather all necessary documentation, such as transcripts or proof of employment, to support your application.

It's also essential to be aware of the application fees. The cost of the PTCB exam is an investment in your professional future, and understanding the financial commitment involved is part of the preparation process. Fee structures are clearly outlined on the PTCB website, and it's a good idea to review these details to ensure you're fully informed.

After submitting your application, the PTCB will review your information to verify that you meet all eligibility requirements. This review process is thorough, ensuring that all candidates are qualified to sit for the exam. Once your application is approved, you'll receive an authorization to schedule your exam. This authorization is a significant milestone, bringing you one step closer to certification. The next phase involves scheduling your exam at a Pearson VUE test center. Pearson VUE administers the PTCE and provides numerous testing locations across the country. This flexibility allows you to choose a test center that is convenient for you, minimizing travel time and stress on exam day. When scheduling your exam, consider your preparation timeline and select a date that gives you ample time to study and review the material.

Preparing for the PTCB exam requires a strategic approach. Utilize the study plan you've developed, incorporating a mix of study methods and resources to cover all exam domains thoroughly. The eligibility criteria you've met—whether through education, training, or work experience—have already provided you with a solid foundation. Now, it's about building on that foundation, deepening your knowledge, and honing your skills.

As you prepare, keep in mind the importance of ethical behavior and professionalism, which are core to the pharmacy technician role. The PTCB exam not only tests your knowledge but also assesses your understanding of the ethical standards that govern the profession. Reflect on your experiences, consider the ethical dilemmas you may face in practice, and think about how you would handle them. This reflection will serve you well, both on the exam and in your future career.

In addition to studying the technical content, consider incorporating exam-taking strategies into your preparation. Familiarize yourself with the format of the PTCE, practice with sample questions, and simulate exam conditions to build your confidence. Time management is crucial during the exam, so practice pacing yourself to ensure you can complete all questions within the allotted time.

The PTCB exam is a significant step in your professional journey, and understanding the eligibility criteria is the first key to unlocking this opportunity. Whether you've completed a formal training program, gained valuable work experience, or both, your path to eligibility reflects your dedication and commitment to the pharmacy technician profession. By meeting these criteria, you've demonstrated that you have the foundational knowledge and skills necessary to succeed.

Now, with your eligibility confirmed, you can focus on the next stages of preparation and exam scheduling. Embrace this journey with confidence and determination, knowing that each step brings you closer to achieving your goal of becoming a certified pharmacy technician. The knowledge and experience you've gained thus far are your tools for success, and with the right preparation and mindset, you are well on your way to passing the PTCB exam and advancing your career in pharmacy.

Navigating the registration process for the Pharmacy Technician Certification Exam (PTCE) might seem daunting at first, but with a clear, step-by-step approach, you'll find it manageable and straightforward. This guide will walk you through each phase of registration, ensuring you're well-prepared and confident as you take this important step towards certification.

The first step in your registration journey is to visit the Pharmacy Technician Certification Board (PTCB) website. This online portal is your primary resource for all things related to the exam, from eligibility requirements to study materials and, of course, the registration process. Start by creating an account on the PTCB website if you don't already have one. This account will be your central hub for managing your application, exam scheduling, and tracking your certification status.

To create an account, navigate to the PTCB homepage and look for the registration or sign-up link. Click on it and follow the prompts to enter your personal information, including your name, email address, and a secure password. Make sure the details you provide match the identification you'll present on exam day, as discrepancies can cause complications. Once your account is set up, you'll receive a confirmation email. Click the link in the email to verify your account and complete the initial registration step.

With your account created and verified, log in to access the candidate dashboard. This is where you'll find the application form for the PTCE. The application requires detailed information about your educational background, training, and work experience. Gather all necessary documents beforehand, such as transcripts, diplomas, and employment verification letters, to streamline this process.

Begin by filling out your personal information. Ensure accuracy and completeness, as errors can delay your application. Next, provide details about your education. If you've completed a formal pharmacy technician training program, include the institution's name, your dates of attendance, and any credentials received. For those qualifying through work experience, describe your role, the name and location of your employer, and the duration of your employment. Be as specific as possible to give a clear picture of your qualifications.

The application also includes sections on your criminal background and any actions taken against your professional license or registration. Full disclosure is crucial here; honesty is the best policy, and the PTCB will verify the information you provide. If you have any concerns about past incidents, it's advisable to contact the PTCB directly for guidance.

Once you've completed the application form, review all your entries carefully. Double-check for typos, missing information, or inconsistencies. When you're confident everything is correct, submit your application. You'll then be prompted to pay the exam fee. The fee for the PTCE is an investment in your professional future, and payment can usually be made via credit card or other electronic payment methods.

After submitting your application and fee, the PTCB will review your submission. This review process ensures all candidates meet the necessary eligibility requirements. Typically, you'll receive a response within a few weeks. During this waiting period, it's a good idea to continue your exam preparation, keeping your study momentum going.

Once your application is approved, you'll receive an Authorization to Test (ATT) email from the PTCB. This email contains important information, including your authorization number and instructions for scheduling your exam. Keep this email safe, as you'll need the details to book your test appointment.

With your ATT in hand, it's time to schedule your exam. The PTCE is administered by Pearson VUE, a leading provider of computer-based testing. Visit the Pearson VUE website and create an account if you don't already have one. Log in to your account, enter your authorization number, and select the Pharmacy Technician Certification Exam from the list of available tests.

Next, choose a test center location that is convenient for you. Pearson VUE has numerous testing centers across the country, so you should be able to find one within a reasonable distance. Consider factors such as travel time and accessibility when making your selection. Once you've chosen a location, select a date and time for your exam. Pick a date that gives you ample time to review and prepare, but also fits within the validity period of your ATT, which is typically 90 days.

After scheduling your exam, you'll receive a confirmation email from Pearson VUE. This email will include the details of your test appointment, such as the date, time, and location. Review this information carefully to ensure everything is correct. If you need to reschedule or cancel your appointment, be aware of the policies and deadlines to avoid any additional fees or complications.

As your exam date approaches, make sure you're familiar with the test center's rules and procedures. On exam day, arrive at the test center at least 30 minutes early to allow time for check-in. Bring two forms of valid identification, one of which must be a government-issued photo ID. The names on your IDs must match the name you used during registration. Personal belongings, including electronic devices and study materials, are not allowed in the testing area, so plan accordingly. The test center will provide a locker to store your items.

During the check-in process, you'll be asked to sign in, have your photo taken, and provide a digital signature. You may also undergo a security check to ensure you're not bringing any prohibited items into the exam room. Once checked in, you'll be escorted to a computer workstation and given a brief tutorial on how to navigate the exam interface.

The PTCE consists of 90 multiple-choice questions, and you'll have two hours to complete the exam. The test is designed to evaluate your knowledge and skills across several key domains of pharmacy practice. Stay calm and focused, and manage your time effectively. If you encounter a difficult question, make an educated guess and move on, returning to it later if time permits.

Upon completing the exam, you'll receive an unofficial score report indicating whether you passed or failed. The official score report will be available in your PTCB account within a few weeks. If you pass, congratulations! You'll receive your certification and can begin using the CPhT (Certified Pharmacy Technician) credential. If you do not pass, don't be discouraged. Use the experience to identify areas for improvement, and prepare to retake the exam.

In conclusion, registering for the PTCB exam is a step-by-step process that requires careful attention to detail and thorough preparation. By following this guide, you can navigate the registration with confidence, ensuring you meet all requirements and are well-prepared for exam day. Remember, each step brings you closer to achieving your goal of becoming a certified pharmacy technician, and with determination and dedication, success is within your reach.

UNDERSTANDING THE PTCB EXAM FORMAT

Grasping the format of the PTCB exam is pivotal for your preparation strategy. Knowing what to expect not only boosts your confidence but also helps you plan your study sessions more effectively. The Pharmacy Technician Certification Exam (PTCE) is designed to assess your knowledge and skills across various domains of pharmacy practice, ensuring you're ready to perform competently as a pharmacy technician.

The PTCE consists of 90 multiple-choice questions, but it's important to note that not all questions are scored. Out of these 90 questions, 80 are scored, and 10 are unscored. The unscored questions are pretest items that the PTCB is evaluating for future exams. Although these unscored questions don't affect your final score, they are mixed in with the scored questions, and you won't know which ones they are. This structure ensures a robust and reliable testing process, but it means you need to treat every question with equal seriousness.

The exam is administered via computer at Pearson VUE test centers, which are equipped with the necessary technology to provide a seamless testing experience. When you arrive at the test center, you'll go through a check-in process that includes presenting identification and securing your personal belongings. You'll be guided to a workstation where you'll take the exam on a computer. Before starting the test, you'll have the opportunity to complete a brief tutorial on how to navigate the exam interface. This tutorial is not part of the exam time, so take advantage of it to familiarize yourself with the system.

You'll have two hours to complete the PTCE. This timeframe includes the time spent on the 90 questions and any breaks you might need. Managing your time effectively is crucial. With 120 minutes available, you have an average of 1.33 minutes per question. However, some questions may take longer than others, so it's essential to pace yourself. If you encounter a challenging question, it's often best to make a note of it, move on, and return to it later if time permits. This strategy helps maintain your momentum and ensures you answer as many questions as possible.

The questions themselves are designed to assess knowledge across four primary domains: Medications, Federal Requirements, Patient Safety and Quality Assurance, and Order Entry and Processing. Each domain represents critical areas of pharmacy practice that are essential for a pharmacy technician to master.

The Medications domain is the most substantial, comprising about 40% of the exam. This section tests your knowledge of drug classifications, generic and brand names, side effects, interactions, and proper dosing. Understanding pharmacology is fundamental to your role, as you'll need to accurately dispense medications and provide relevant information to patients.

Federal Requirements make up approximately 12.5% of the exam. This domain covers the legal aspects of pharmacy practice, including the Controlled Substances Act, the Food, Drug, and

Cosmetic Act, and other federal regulations. Familiarity with these laws is essential for ensuring compliance and maintaining patient safety.

Patient Safety and Quality Assurance accounts for about 26.25% of the exam. This section focuses on practices and protocols that ensure the safety and well-being of patients. Topics include error prevention strategies, proper medication storage and handling, and quality control measures. Your ability to implement these practices is critical for minimizing risks and ensuring high standards of care.

Order Entry and Processing constitutes around 21.25% of the exam. This domain evaluates your skills in interpreting prescriptions, entering orders into the pharmacy system, and ensuring the accuracy of medication dispensing. Efficient and accurate order processing is vital for maintaining workflow and preventing errors that could impact patient health.

Each question on the PTCE is a multiple-choice question with four possible answers. Only one answer is correct, so it's important to read each question carefully and consider all options before selecting your answer. Sometimes, eliminating the obviously incorrect answers first can help you narrow down your choices and increase your chances of selecting the correct one.

In addition to understanding the content and structure of the questions, it's also beneficial to familiarize yourself with the types of questions you might encounter. The PTCE includes a mix of straightforward recall questions, which test your ability to remember specific facts, and application questions, which require you to apply your knowledge to real-world scenarios. For example, you might be asked to identify a drug based on its classification or to determine the correct course of action in a particular pharmacy situation.

As you prepare for the exam, practice tests can be an invaluable resource. They not only help you get used to the format of the questions but also allow you to gauge your knowledge and identify areas where you need further study. When taking practice tests, simulate exam conditions by timing yourself and working in a quiet environment. This practice helps build your test-taking stamina and improves your ability to manage time effectively.

On exam day, staying calm and focused is key. Anxiety is natural, but it's important to keep it in check to maintain clarity of thought. Deep breathing exercises and positive visualization can help manage stress. Remember, the preparation you've done has equipped you with the knowledge and skills you need to succeed.

During the exam, keep an eye on the clock, but don't let it dominate your thoughts. If you find yourself spending too much time on a single question, it's better to move on and come back to it later. This approach helps ensure that you have time to answer all the questions.

Once you've completed the exam, take a moment to review your answers if time allows. Check for any questions you may have skipped and ensure that all your answers are properly recorded. When you're satisfied, submit your exam and take a deep breath. You've completed an important step towards your certification.

In conclusion, understanding the PTCB exam format is crucial for effective preparation. Knowing what to expect helps you approach the exam with confidence and clarity. From the structure of the questions to the content domains, every aspect of the PTCE is designed to evaluate your readiness to be a certified pharmacy technician. By familiarizing yourself with the format and practicing under realistic conditions, you can optimize your study efforts and enhance your performance on exam day. Remember, thorough preparation and a calm, focused approach will guide you to success.

WHAT TO EXPECT ON THE DAY OF THE EXAM

The day of the Pharmacy Technician Certification Exam (PTCE) has finally arrived. After all your diligent preparation and hard work, it's natural to feel a mix of excitement and anxiety. Knowing what to expect can help you manage these emotions and approach the exam with confidence and clarity. Let's walk through the key aspects of exam day, from the moment you wake up to the time you leave the test center, equipped with the knowledge that you've done your best.

Start your day with a good breakfast. Opt for something that will give you sustained energy, such as whole grains, protein, and fruits. Avoid heavy, greasy foods that might make you feel sluggish. A balanced meal will help maintain your focus and stamina throughout the exam. Stay hydrated, but be mindful not to overdo it to avoid frequent bathroom breaks during the test.

As you get ready, double-check that you have all necessary documents and materials. You'll need two forms of valid identification, one of which must be a government-issued photo ID. Ensure that the name on your IDs matches the name you used to register for the exam. Familiarize yourself with the testing center's address and plan your route in advance. Aim to arrive at least 30 minutes early to account for any unexpected delays, such as traffic or parking difficulties.

Dressing comfortably is important. Choose layers that you can easily add or remove, as testing centers can vary in temperature. Comfort is key to minimizing distractions and keeping your focus on the exam.

When you arrive at the test center, you'll first check in at the reception area. The staff will verify your identification and provide instructions for storing personal belongings. Typically, you'll be assigned a locker to secure items like bags, phones, and jackets. Only bring essentials to the test center to streamline this process.

After securing your belongings, you'll proceed to the testing area. Here, you may undergo a security check, which can include scanning with a metal detector wand and a brief pat-down. This step ensures the integrity of the testing environment. Once cleared, you'll be guided to a computer workstation.

Before the exam begins, you'll have an opportunity to complete a short tutorial on the testing interface. This tutorial will show you how to navigate through the questions, use the on-screen calculator, and mark questions for review. This time does not count towards your two-hour exam limit, so take advantage of it to familiarize yourself with the system. Completing the tutorial helps reduce any initial anxiety and ensures you're comfortable with the tools available.

As the exam starts, take a deep breath and focus. The PTCE consists of 90 multiple-choice questions, including 10 unscored pretest questions. You'll have 120 minutes to complete the exam, which means you should pace yourself. On average, you have about 1.33 minutes per question. However, some questions will be easier and quicker to answer than others. If you encounter a challenging question, don't get stuck. Mark it for review, make your best guess, and move on. You can always come back to it later if you have time.

The exam covers four main domains: Medications, Federal Requirements, Patient Safety and Quality Assurance, and Order Entry and Processing. Each question is designed to test your knowledge and ability to apply it in real-world scenarios. Stay calm and read each question carefully, ensuring you understand what is being asked before selecting your answer. Use the process of elimination to narrow down your choices, and trust your preparation.

During the exam, maintain awareness of the time without letting it dominate your thoughts. The exam interface usually includes a timer, so you can check how much time you have left. It's a good strategy to periodically glance at the timer to ensure you're on track. If you find yourself ahead of schedule, use the extra time to review your answers and revisit any marked questions.

If you need a break, you can take one, but the clock will continue to run. Therefore, keep breaks brief. Stretching and deep breathing can help rejuvenate you without taking too much time away from the exam. Remember, it's better to take a short break and return refreshed than to struggle through fatigue or anxiety.

Once you complete the exam, you'll have a chance to review your answers if time permits. Use this opportunity to revisit any questions you were unsure about and make any necessary changes. Trust your instincts but also reconsider any flagged questions with a fresh perspective.

After submitting your exam, you'll receive an unofficial score report. This immediate feedback lets you know if you've passed or not. The official results will be available in your PTCB account within a few weeks. If you pass, congratulations! You've earned your certification and can proudly use the CPhT credential. If you don't pass, take some time to reflect on your experience. Identify areas for improvement, and use this insight to prepare for a retake.

Leaving the test center, take a moment to acknowledge your hard work and dedication. Regardless of the outcome, you've reached a significant milestone in your journey. If you passed, celebrate your achievement and start planning your next steps as a certified pharmacy technician. If you need to retake the exam, stay positive and focused. Use the experience to strengthen your knowledge and approach the next attempt with renewed determination.

In conclusion, knowing what to expect on the day of the PTCE can greatly enhance your confidence and performance. From a healthy start to the day to understanding the test center procedures and managing your time during the exam, each aspect plays a crucial role in your success. By staying calm, prepared, and focused, you can navigate the exam day with ease and achieve your goal of becoming a certified pharmacy technician. Remember, this is a significant step towards a rewarding career, and your preparation and perseverance will pay off.

3. FUNDAMENTAL KNOWLEDGE

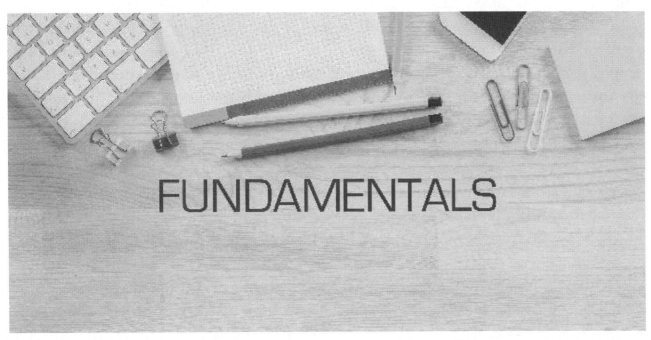

Diving into the world of pharmacy requires a solid foundation of fundamental knowledge. This chapter is your gateway to the essential concepts and principles that underpin the practice of pharmacy. Understanding the basics of pharmacology, the intricacies of drug classes, and the protocols for dispensing medications forms the bedrock of your expertise as a pharmacy technician.

Imagine stepping into a pharmacy for the first time, surrounded by shelves lined with medications. Each bottle and box represents a wealth of information about chemistry, biology, and patient care. Your ability to navigate this landscape with confidence depends on mastering the core knowledge presented in this chapter. We will explore key drug classifications, the mechanisms of action, and the therapeutic uses of various medications.

Additionally, we'll delve into the crucial aspects of federal and state pharmacy laws, ensuring you comprehend the legal framework that guides your professional actions. Ethics and privacy in pharmacy practice are also paramount, safeguarding the trust patients place in you.

By the end of this chapter, you'll be equipped with the foundational knowledge necessary to support your role and advance your career in pharmacy. Let's embark on this educational journey together, laying the groundwork for your future success.

INTRODUCTION TO PHARMACOLOGY BASICS

Understanding the basics of pharmacology is akin to unlocking the door to the intricate world of medications and their impact on the human body. As a pharmacy technician, having a firm grasp of these fundamentals is essential, as it forms the backbone of your professional knowledge and allows you to assist pharmacists effectively and safely. Let's delve into the key principles of pharmacology, exploring how drugs work, their classifications, and their interactions with the body.

At its core, pharmacology is the science of drugs, encompassing their origins, composition, pharmacokinetics, pharmacodynamics, therapeutic uses, and potential side effects. To navigate this complex field, we start with the foundational concepts of pharmacokinetics and pharmacodynamics.

Pharmacokinetics describes what the body does to a drug. It involves four main processes: absorption, distribution, metabolism, and excretion, often remembered by the acronym ADME.

- **Absorption** is the process by which a drug enters the bloodstream. This can happen through various routes such as oral, intravenous, intramuscular, subcutaneous, and topical. Each route has its own absorption characteristics, influencing how quickly and effectively a drug begins to work. For instance, intravenous administration allows for immediate absorption into the bloodstream, while oral medications must pass through the digestive system, affecting the onset of action.

- **Distribution** refers to the dispersion of a drug throughout the body fluids and tissues. The extent and pattern of distribution depend on factors such as blood flow, tissue permeability, and the drug's affinity for different tissues. Drugs often bind to plasma proteins, which can affect their free (active) concentration in the bloodstream.

- **Metabolism**, primarily occurring in the liver, involves the chemical alteration of the drug. This process transforms the drug into metabolites, which can be either active or inactive. The liver's enzymes, particularly the cytochrome P450 family, play a crucial role in drug metabolism. Understanding these metabolic pathways helps predict drug interactions and the potential for side effects.

- **Excretion** is the removal of the drug and its metabolites from the body, primarily through the kidneys (urine) and, to a lesser extent, through bile (feces), sweat, saliva, and breath. The rate of excretion affects the drug's duration of action and is a key factor in determining appropriate dosing intervals.

Pharmacodynamics, on the other hand, explains what the drug does to the body. It involves the mechanisms of drug action and the relationship between drug concentration and effect.

- Drugs typically exert their effects by binding to specific cellular receptors, enzymes, or ion channels. This interaction can either stimulate (agonist) or inhibit (antagonist) the receptor's natural action. For example, beta-blockers are antagonists that inhibit the effects of adrenaline on beta receptors, reducing heart rate and blood pressure.

- The dose-response relationship is a critical concept in pharmacodynamics. It describes how the magnitude of a drug's effect changes with its concentration. Understanding this relationship helps in determining the optimal dose that achieves the desired therapeutic effect while minimizing adverse effects.

Drugs are classified into various categories based on their therapeutic effects, chemical characteristics, and mechanisms of action. Common classifications include:

- **Analgesics**, which relieve pain (e.g., acetaminophen, ibuprofen)
- **Antibiotics**, which treat bacterial infections (e.g., amoxicillin, ciprofloxacin)
- **Antihypertensives**, which lower blood pressure (e.g., lisinopril, amlodipine)
- **Antidiabetics**, which manage diabetes (e.g., metformin, insulin)

- **Antidepressants**, which treat depression (e.g., fluoxetine, sertraline)

Each drug class has its own set of indications, mechanisms, and potential side effects, necessitating a thorough understanding to ensure safe and effective use.

Drug interactions are another critical aspect of pharmacology. These interactions can enhance or diminish a drug's effects and can be classified into three main types:

- **Drug-drug interactions** occur when two or more drugs influence each other's effects. For example, combining a blood thinner like warfarin with an anti-inflammatory drug like aspirin can increase the risk of bleeding.
- **Drug-food interactions** happen when certain foods affect a drug's absorption or metabolism. A well-known example is the interaction between grapefruit juice and statins, where the juice inhibits the metabolism of the drug, leading to increased blood levels and potential toxicity.
- **Drug-disease interactions** are when a drug exacerbates an existing medical condition. For instance, nonsteroidal anti-inflammatory drugs (NSAIDs) can worsen hypertension and should be used cautiously in patients with high blood pressure.

Understanding these interactions helps prevent adverse effects and ensures that medications work as intended.

Side effects, or adverse drug reactions, are unwanted effects that occur at normal drug dosages. They can range from mild (nausea, headache) to severe (allergic reactions, liver damage). Being aware of common side effects and monitoring patients for these reactions is an integral part of pharmacy practice.

Ethical considerations in pharmacology are also paramount. Ensuring patient safety, maintaining confidentiality, and providing accurate information about medications are responsibilities that pharmacy technicians must uphold. This ethical framework guides your actions and decisions, ensuring that patient care remains the top priority.

As you progress in your career, continuing education in pharmacology will be crucial. The field is dynamic, with ongoing research leading to new drugs, updated guidelines, and evolving therapeutic practices. Staying informed through professional development opportunities, such as workshops, courses, and conferences, will help you maintain your expertise and provide the best possible care to patients.

In summary, an introduction to pharmacology basics equips you with essential knowledge about how drugs interact with the body and how the body affects drugs. From pharmacokinetics and pharmacodynamics to drug classifications and interactions, these fundamentals are the building blocks of your pharmacy education. As you delve deeper into this field, you'll gain the skills and understanding necessary to support pharmacists and ensure the safe, effective use of medications. This foundational knowledge not only prepares you for the PTCE but also sets the stage for a successful and impactful career in pharmacy.

OVERVIEW OF KEY DRUG CLASSES

The world of pharmacy is vast and diverse, with countless medications designed to treat a myriad of conditions. To navigate this complex landscape effectively, it's essential to understand the key drug classes, each defined by specific therapeutic effects and mechanisms of action. This knowledge not only aids in your day-to-day tasks but also ensures you can provide accurate information and support to both pharmacists and patients. Let's embark on an exploration of these fundamental drug classes, highlighting their primary uses, mechanisms, and notable examples.

Analgesics

Analgesics are drugs designed to relieve pain without causing loss of consciousness. They are divided into two main categories: non-opioid and opioid analgesics.

- **Non-opioid analgesics**, such as acetaminophen and nonsteroidal anti-inflammatory drugs (NSAIDs) like ibuprofen and aspirin, work by inhibiting the synthesis of prostaglandins, substances that mediate inflammation and pain. These drugs are commonly used for mild to moderate pain, fever reduction, and inflammation control.
- **Opioid analgesics**, such as morphine, oxycodone, and hydrocodone, act on the central nervous system by binding to opioid receptors, which block the transmission of pain signals to the brain. They are used for moderate to severe pain but come with a higher risk of dependence and side effects such as respiratory depression, constipation, and sedation.

Antibiotics

Antibiotics are agents that kill or inhibit the growth of bacteria, essential in treating bacterial infections. They are classified based on their mechanism of action and the type of bacteria they target.

- **Beta-lactams**, including penicillins (amoxicillin) and cephalosporins (ceftriaxone), disrupt bacterial cell wall synthesis, leading to cell lysis and death. They are effective against a broad range of bacterial infections.
- **Macrolides**, like azithromycin and erythromycin, inhibit bacterial protein synthesis by binding to the ribosomal subunit. They are often used for respiratory tract infections and skin infections.
- **Quinolones**, such as ciprofloxacin and levofloxacin, inhibit bacterial DNA gyrase and topoisomerase IV, enzymes critical for DNA replication. They are used to treat urinary tract infections, gastrointestinal infections, and some types of pneumonia.
- **Aminoglycosides**, like gentamicin and tobramycin, also inhibit protein synthesis but are typically reserved for severe infections due to their potential for nephrotoxicity and ototoxicity.

Antihypertensives

Antihypertensives are used to manage high blood pressure, reducing the risk of cardiovascular events such as stroke and heart attack. They encompass several classes, each targeting different pathways to lower blood pressure.

- **ACE inhibitors** (angiotensin-converting enzyme inhibitors), such as lisinopril and enalapril, prevent the conversion of angiotensin I to angiotensin II, a potent vasoconstrictor. This results in vasodilation and reduced blood pressure.

- **ARBs** (angiotensin II receptor blockers), like losartan and valsartan, block the action of angiotensin II, offering a similar effect to ACE inhibitors but with a lower risk of cough, a common side effect of ACE inhibitors.
- **Calcium channel blockers**, such as amlodipine and diltiazem, inhibit calcium ion influx into cardiac and smooth muscle cells, leading to relaxation of blood vessels and decreased blood pressure. They are also used for certain types of arrhythmias.
- **Beta-blockers**, like metoprolol and atenolol, reduce blood pressure by blocking beta-adrenergic receptors, decreasing heart rate and cardiac output. They are also used for angina, heart failure, and arrhythmias.
- **Diuretics**, such as hydrochlorothiazide and furosemide, promote the excretion of sodium and water from the body, reducing blood volume and pressure. They are often used in combination with other antihypertensives.

Antidiabetics

Antidiabetics help manage blood glucose levels in individuals with diabetes. They are broadly classified into oral hypoglycemics and injectable insulin.

- **Biguanides**, with metformin being the most notable example, reduce hepatic glucose production and improve insulin sensitivity. They are the first-line treatment for type 2 diabetes.
- **Sulfonylureas**, such as glipizide and glyburide, stimulate pancreatic beta cells to release more insulin. They are effective but can cause hypoglycemia, especially in older adults.
- **DPP-4 inhibitors** (dipeptidyl peptidase-4 inhibitors), like sitagliptin and saxagliptin, enhance the body's incretin system, which increases insulin release and decreases glucagon levels post-meal.
- **GLP-1 agonists** (glucagon-like peptide-1 agonists), such as liraglutide and exenatide, also enhance incretin activity but are injectable. They promote insulin release, inhibit glucagon release, and slow gastric emptying.
- **Insulin** is used primarily in type 1 diabetes but also in type 2 diabetes when oral medications are insufficient. It comes in various forms, including rapid-acting (lispro), short-acting (regular insulin), intermediate-acting (NPH), and long-acting (glargine).

Antidepressants

Antidepressants treat depression and other mood disorders by altering neurotransmitter levels in the brain.

- **SSRIs** (selective serotonin reuptake inhibitors), such as fluoxetine and sertraline, increase serotonin levels by inhibiting its reuptake into presynaptic cells. They are commonly used due to their efficacy and relatively mild side effect profile.
- **SNRIs** (serotonin-norepinephrine reuptake inhibitors), like venlafaxine and duloxetine, increase levels of both serotonin and norepinephrine. They are used for depression, anxiety disorders, and chronic pain conditions.

- **TCAs** (tricyclic antidepressants), such as amitriptyline and nortriptyline, block the reuptake of serotonin and norepinephrine but have a broader side effect profile, including anticholinergic effects and cardiotoxicity.
- **MAOIs** (monoamine oxidase inhibitors), like phenelzine and tranylcypromine, inhibit the enzyme monoamine oxidase, which breaks down neurotransmitters like serotonin, norepinephrine, and dopamine. They are effective but require dietary restrictions due to potentially severe interactions with tyramine-containing foods.

Antipsychotics

Antipsychotics are used to manage psychosis, including schizophrenia and bipolar disorder. They are divided into typical (first-generation) and atypical (second-generation) antipsychotics.

- **Typical antipsychotics**, such as haloperidol and chlorpromazine, primarily block dopamine receptors, which can reduce psychotic symptoms but also cause extrapyramidal side effects (movement disorders).
- **Atypical antipsychotics**, like risperidone and olanzapine, target both dopamine and serotonin receptors. They tend to have a lower risk of movement disorders but can cause metabolic side effects like weight gain and diabetes.

Anticoagulants

Anticoagulants prevent blood clot formation, reducing the risk of stroke and other thrombotic events.

- **Warfarin** is a vitamin K antagonist that reduces the synthesis of clotting factors. It requires regular blood monitoring (INR) and has numerous dietary and drug interactions.
- **Direct oral anticoagulants (DOACs)**, such as rivaroxaban, apixaban, and dabigatran, provide a more predictable anticoagulant effect without the need for regular monitoring. They inhibit specific clotting factors like factor Xa or thrombin.

Bronchodilators

Bronchodilators are used to relieve bronchospasm in conditions like asthma and chronic obstructive pulmonary disease (COPD).

- **Beta-agonists**, such as albuterol and salmeterol, relax bronchial smooth muscle by stimulating beta-2 adrenergic receptors. Short-acting beta-agonists (SABAs) provide quick relief, while long-acting beta-agonists (LABAs) are used for maintenance therapy.
- **Anticholinergics**, like ipratropium and tiotropium, block muscarinic receptors in the airways, reducing bronchoconstriction. They are often used in combination with beta-agonists for enhanced effect.

Understanding these key drug classes is fundamental to your role as a pharmacy technician. Each class has its unique characteristics, therapeutic uses, and potential side effects. Familiarity with these details not only enhances your ability to support pharmacists but also ensures you can provide accurate and safe information to patients. As you continue to build on this foundational knowledge, you'll be better equipped to navigate the complexities of pharmacy practice and contribute meaningfully to patient care.

Mastering the protocols and procedures in dispensing medications is a critical aspect of your role as a pharmacy technician. This involves a combination of accuracy, attention to detail, and adherence to regulatory guidelines to ensure patient safety and effective treatment. Let's delve into the essential steps and best practices that define the dispensing process, from receiving a prescription to handing over the medication to the patient.

Receiving and Interpreting Prescriptions

The dispensing process begins with receiving a prescription, whether electronically, in writing, or verbally. Each type of prescription requires careful scrutiny to ensure it meets all necessary legal and professional standards.

For written prescriptions, verify the presence of key information: the patient's name, date of birth, the date the prescription was written, the name and strength of the medication, dosage instructions, quantity, and the prescriber's signature. Electronic prescriptions, which are becoming increasingly common, are typically transmitted directly from the prescriber's office to the pharmacy's computer system. These also need verification for completeness and accuracy.

When interpreting a prescription, clarity is crucial. Any ambiguity in the prescription details, such as unclear handwriting or unusual dosage instructions, should prompt immediate clarification from the prescriber. This prevents potential medication errors and ensures the patient receives the correct treatment.

Entering Prescription Information

Once the prescription is verified, the next step is to enter the details into the pharmacy's information system. This step involves accurately inputting the patient's information, medication name, dosage, instructions, and any other relevant details into the system. Precision here is vital as errors can lead to significant adverse outcomes.

Double-check the entered information against the original prescription to ensure accuracy. Modern pharmacy information systems often include safeguards such as drug interaction alerts and dosage checks, which provide an additional layer of safety by flagging potential issues.

Selecting and Measuring the Medication

With the prescription information entered, the next task is to select the correct medication. This step requires thorough knowledge of medication names, both generic and brand, as well as their physical characteristics. Confirm that the medication selected matches the prescription in terms of drug name, strength, and dosage form (e.g., tablet, capsule, liquid).

Measuring the correct quantity of medication is equally important. For tablets and capsules, this involves counting the exact number prescribed. Automated pill counters are commonly used to enhance accuracy and efficiency, but manual counting is still required in some settings, necessitating meticulous attention to detail.

For liquid medications, precise measurement using appropriate tools such as graduated cylinders or dosing syringes ensures the patient receives the correct dose. Reconstitution of powdered medications requires following specific instructions to mix the medication with the correct amount of diluent, achieving the desired concentration.

Labeling and Packaging

Labeling the medication correctly is another critical step in the dispensing process. The label must include the patient's name, medication name, strength, dosage instructions, quantity, prescriber's name, the pharmacy's contact information, and any relevant warnings or instructions. This label serves as a vital communication tool between the pharmacy and the patient, ensuring proper usage and adherence to the prescribed regimen.

In addition to the primary label, auxiliary labels are often used to provide additional information such as storage instructions ("Refrigerate"), usage warnings ("May cause drowsiness"), or specific administration instructions ("Take with food"). These labels enhance patient safety and compliance by highlighting important aspects of medication use.

Packaging the medication appropriately is also essential. For solid medications like tablets and capsules, child-resistant containers are typically used to prevent accidental ingestion. Liquid medications may require specific types of bottles or dosing devices to ensure accurate administration. The packaging must be secure, protecting the medication from contamination and degradation.

Pharmacist Verification

Before the medication is dispensed to the patient, it undergoes a final verification by the pharmacist. This step is a critical safety checkpoint. The pharmacist reviews the entire dispensing process, ensuring that the right medication, in the correct dosage and quantity, has been prepared according to the prescription. They also check for potential drug interactions, contraindications, and patient-specific factors that might affect medication efficacy and safety.

During this verification, the pharmacist may also review the patient's medication history and provide counseling on new medications or changes to existing therapy. This interaction is an opportunity to educate the patient about their treatment, answer questions, and reinforce the importance of adherence to the prescribed regimen.

Patient Consultation and Medication Delivery

The final step in the dispensing process is delivering the medication to the patient and providing necessary consultation. Effective communication here is key to ensuring the patient understands how to use their medication correctly and safely. This consultation should cover several important points:

1. **Medication Name and Purpose:** Explain what the medication is called and why it has been prescribed.
2. **Dosage and Administration:** Provide clear instructions on how to take the medication, including the dosage, timing, and any special instructions (e.g., "Take with food").
3. **Duration of Therapy:** Inform the patient how long they should take the medication and what to do if they miss a dose.
4. **Potential Side Effects:** Discuss common side effects and what to do if they occur. Provide guidance on when to seek medical attention for more serious reactions.

5. **Storage Instructions:** Advise on how to store the medication properly to maintain its efficacy (e.g., "Keep refrigerated").
6. **Drug Interactions:** Highlight any known interactions with other medications, foods, or supplements the patient is using.

Encourage the patient to ask questions and express any concerns they may have. This dialogue not only empowers the patient but also helps identify and address potential issues that could affect medication adherence and outcomes.

Documentation and Record Keeping

Maintaining accurate and comprehensive records is a fundamental aspect of the dispensing process. Documentation includes recording the prescription details, any communications with the prescriber, and notes from the patient consultation. This information is crucial for ongoing patient care, enabling continuity and coordination among healthcare providers.

Pharmacy records must be kept in compliance with regulatory requirements, ensuring they are secure, confidential, and accessible when needed. These records support quality assurance processes, audits, and legal obligations, contributing to the overall safety and efficiency of pharmacy operations.

Continuous Quality Improvement

Dispensing protocols and procedures are not static; they evolve with advancements in pharmacy practice, technology, and regulatory standards. Continuous quality improvement (CQI) programs are essential for identifying and addressing errors, enhancing workflows, and improving patient outcomes.

Pharmacy technicians play a vital role in CQI by reporting errors or near misses, participating in training and education programs, and contributing to the development of best practices. Embracing a culture of continuous improvement ensures that the dispensing process remains safe, efficient, and patient-centered.

In conclusion, mastering the protocols and procedures in dispensing is fundamental to your role as a pharmacy technician. From receiving and interpreting prescriptions to patient consultation and documentation, each step requires meticulous attention to detail and a commitment to patient safety. By following these best practices and continuously striving for excellence, you contribute to the effective delivery of healthcare and the well-being of your patients. This comprehensive understanding of the dispensing process not only prepares you for the PTCE but also equips you with the skills and knowledge necessary for a successful career in pharmacy.

FEDERAL PHARMACY LAWS AND HOW THEY AFFECT YOU

Navigating the world of pharmacy involves not only understanding medications but also being well-versed in the federal laws that govern pharmacy practice. These laws are designed to ensure the safe and effective use of medications, protect public health, and maintain the integrity of the pharmacy profession. As a pharmacy technician, knowing these laws and how they affect your daily responsibilities is crucial. Let's explore the key federal pharmacy laws and their implications for your role.

The Controlled Substances Act (CSA)

One of the most significant pieces of legislation affecting pharmacy practice is the Controlled Substances Act (CSA). Enacted in 1970, the CSA regulates the manufacture, distribution, and dispensing of controlled substances, categorizing drugs into five schedules based on their potential for abuse and accepted medical use.

- **Schedule I** drugs have a high potential for abuse and no accepted medical use in the United States. Examples include heroin, LSD, and ecstasy. These substances are not available for prescribing and are strictly controlled for research purposes only.
- **Schedule II** drugs have a high potential for abuse but have accepted medical uses with severe restrictions. Examples include oxycodone, fentanyl, and methamphetamine. Prescriptions for Schedule II drugs cannot be refilled and require a new prescription for each dispensation.
- **Schedule III** drugs have a lower potential for abuse compared to Schedules I and II and have accepted medical uses. Examples include anabolic steroids, ketamine, and certain barbiturates. These drugs can be refilled up to five times within six months if authorized by the prescriber.
- **Schedule IV** drugs have a lower potential for abuse than Schedule III drugs and have accepted medical uses. Examples include alprazolam, diazepam, and lorazepam. Like Schedule III drugs, they can be refilled up to five times within six months.
- **Schedule V** drugs have the lowest potential for abuse relative to the other schedules and include medications like cough preparations containing less than 200 milligrams of codeine per 100 milliliters. These drugs may be refilled as authorized by the prescriber.

As a pharmacy technician, your responsibilities under the CSA include maintaining accurate records of controlled substances, ensuring secure storage, and adhering to proper inventory management practices. These measures help prevent diversion and misuse of controlled substances.

The Food, Drug, and Cosmetic Act (FDCA)

The Food, Drug, and Cosmetic Act (FDCA) of 1938 is another cornerstone of federal pharmacy law. The FDCA grants the Food and Drug Administration (FDA) the authority to oversee the safety, efficacy, and security of drugs, medical devices, and cosmetics. Key provisions of the FDCA that affect pharmacy practice include:

- **Drug Approval Process:** The FDCA requires that new drugs undergo rigorous testing and clinical trials to demonstrate safety and efficacy before they can be marketed. This process ensures that medications available to the public meet stringent standards.
- **Labeling Requirements:** The FDCA mandates that drug labels provide clear, accurate information about the medication, including its name, dosage, directions for use, and potential side effects. Accurate labeling is crucial for ensuring that patients understand how to use their medications safely.

- **Adulteration and Misbranding:** The FDCA prohibits the distribution of adulterated or misbranded drugs. Adulteration refers to the contamination or impurity of a drug, while misbranding involves false or misleading labeling. These provisions protect consumers from unsafe or ineffective medications.

In your role, ensuring compliance with FDCA regulations means verifying that medications are properly labeled and stored, checking for recalls, and maintaining vigilance for any signs of adulteration or misbranding.

The Drug Enforcement Administration (DEA) Regulations

The Drug Enforcement Administration (DEA) enforces the CSA and other laws related to controlled substances. The DEA's regulations impact several aspects of pharmacy practice, including registration, recordkeeping, and reporting.

- **Registration:** Pharmacies and practitioners who handle controlled substances must register with the DEA. This registration is a legal requirement and ensures that only authorized entities can prescribe, dispense, or distribute controlled substances.
- **Recordkeeping:** Accurate recordkeeping is essential for compliance with DEA regulations. Pharmacies must maintain detailed records of all transactions involving controlled substances, including receipts, dispensing logs, and inventory records. These records help track the flow of controlled substances and prevent diversion.
- **Reporting:** The DEA requires reporting of significant losses or thefts of controlled substances using DEA Form 106. Prompt reporting is critical for mitigating the risk of diversion and initiating investigations.

Adhering to DEA regulations involves meticulous attention to detail in maintaining records, conducting regular inventory checks, and promptly addressing any discrepancies or issues related to controlled substances.

The Health Insurance Portability and Accountability Act (HIPAA)

HIPAA, enacted in 1996, is primarily known for its provisions related to the protection of patient health information. HIPAA's Privacy Rule and Security Rule establish national standards for safeguarding medical records and other personal health information.

- **Privacy Rule:** The Privacy Rule governs the use and disclosure of protected health information (PHI). It grants patients rights over their health information, including the right to access their records and request corrections. Pharmacies must ensure that PHI is disclosed only for permitted purposes, such as treatment, payment, and healthcare operations.
- **Security Rule:** The Security Rule sets standards for protecting electronic PHI (ePHI). It requires the implementation of administrative, physical, and technical safeguards to ensure the confidentiality, integrity, and availability of ePHI. This includes measures like encryption, access controls, and secure data storage.

As a pharmacy technician, you play a crucial role in maintaining HIPAA compliance. This involves safeguarding patient information, ensuring that conversations about medications are private, and using secure methods to handle electronic data. Understanding HIPAA's provisions helps protect patient privacy and builds trust in the healthcare system.

The Combat Methamphetamine Epidemic Act (CMEA)

The Combat Methamphetamine Epidemic Act (CMEA) of 2005 addresses the illegal production of methamphetamine by regulating the sale of precursor chemicals, such as pseudoephedrine, ephedrine, and phenylpropanolamine. These substances are commonly found in over-the-counter cold and allergy medications.

Key provisions of the CMEA include:

- **Sales Limits:** The CMEA imposes daily and monthly limits on the sale of products containing precursor chemicals. For example, consumers cannot purchase more than 3.6 grams per day or 9 grams per month of pseudoephedrine.
- **Logbook Requirements:** Pharmacies must maintain a logbook of sales, recording the purchaser's name, address, date and time of sale, and the amount of product purchased. The purchaser must also present valid identification and sign the logbook.
- **Storage Requirements:** Products containing precursor chemicals must be stored behind the counter or in a locked cabinet to prevent unauthorized access.

Compliance with the CMEA involves training to ensure understanding of sales limits, maintaining accurate logbooks, and properly storing regulated products. These measures help prevent the diversion of precursor chemicals for illicit drug production.

The Poison Prevention Packaging Act (PPPA)

The Poison Prevention Packaging Act (PPPA) of 1970 mandates the use of child-resistant packaging for certain medications and household products to prevent accidental poisonings. Child-resistant packaging is designed to be difficult for children under five years old to open but accessible to adults. Pharmacies must ensure that medications requiring child-resistant packaging are dispensed in compliant containers unless the patient or prescriber requests non-child-resistant packaging. Understanding the PPPA's requirements helps protect young children from accidental ingestion of harmful substances.

The Affordable Care Act (ACA)

The Affordable Care Act (ACA) of 2010 has several provisions that impact pharmacy practice, including expanded access to healthcare, the promotion of preventive services, and the emphasis on medication therapy management (MTM).

- **Preventive Services:** The ACA requires coverage of preventive services without patient cost-sharing. Pharmacies may play a role in providing or facilitating access to preventive services such as immunizations and screenings.
- **Medication Therapy Management:** The ACA supports the expansion of MTM services, which involve comprehensive reviews of a patient's medications to optimize therapeutic outcomes and reduce the risk of adverse effects. Pharmacy technicians often assist pharmacists in delivering MTM services by gathering medication histories and preparing review documents.

In conclusion, federal pharmacy laws provide a framework that ensures the safe, effective, and ethical practice of pharmacy. As a pharmacy technician, understanding these laws and how they affect your responsibilities is essential for compliance and patient safety. From managing controlled substances under the CSA to protecting patient information under HIPAA, each regulation plays a crucial role in the daily operations of a pharmacy. By adhering to these laws and maintaining a commitment to continuous learning, you contribute to the integrity and professionalism of the pharmacy field.

STATE-SPECIFIC PHARMACY REGULATIONS

While federal pharmacy laws provide a broad framework for safe and effective practice, state-specific regulations add another layer of governance that you must navigate as a pharmacy technician. Each state has its own pharmacy board or regulatory authority responsible for setting rules and standards that reflect the unique needs and circumstances of its population. Understanding these state-specific regulations is crucial for compliance and ensuring the highest level of patient care. Let's explore the essential aspects of these regulations and how they impact your role in pharmacy practice.

Licensing and Certification Requirements

One of the primary areas where state regulations differ is in the licensing and certification requirements for pharmacy technicians. While some states mandate national certification through entities like the Pharmacy Technician Certification Board (PTCB) or the National Healthcareer Association (NHA), others have their own certification processes or may not require certification at all.

For example, California requires pharmacy technicians to be licensed by the California State Board of Pharmacy, which includes passing an exam and completing a pharmacy technician training program. In contrast, states like Pennsylvania do not require state-specific licensing but do encourage national certification. Familiarize yourself with your state's specific requirements to ensure compliance and enhance your professional qualifications.

Continuing Education and Training

Continuing education (CE) is another area governed by state regulations. Many states require pharmacy technicians to complete a certain number of CE hours to maintain their certification or license. These educational activities are designed to ensure that pharmacy technicians stay current with evolving practices, new medications, and advancements in pharmacy technology.

For instance, in Florida, pharmacy technicians must complete 20 hours of continuing education every two years, including specific hours dedicated to pharmacy law and medication errors. On the other hand, Texas requires 20 hours of CE, with at least one hour focusing on Texas-specific pharmacy laws and rules. Keeping track of these requirements and planning your CE activities accordingly helps you remain compliant and knowledgeable in your field.

Scope of Practice

State regulations also define the scope of practice for pharmacy technicians, outlining the tasks they are authorized to perform. This scope can vary significantly between states, influencing the responsibilities you can undertake in a pharmacy setting.

In some states, pharmacy technicians can perform tasks such as compounding medications, administering immunizations, and processing prescriptions without pharmacist oversight, provided they have received appropriate training. For example, in Idaho, pharmacy technicians with advanced training are allowed to administer immunizations. Conversely, in states like New York, the scope of practice is more restricted, requiring direct supervision by a pharmacist for many tasks.

Understanding your state's scope of practice regulations ensures that you operate within legal boundaries and utilize your skills to their fullest extent.

Prescription Processing and Dispensing

The rules governing prescription processing and dispensing can also vary by state. These regulations include specific protocols for handling controlled substances, electronic prescriptions, and medication compounding.

For controlled substances, states may have additional requirements beyond federal DEA regulations. For instance, in New York, the Internet System for Tracking Over-Prescribing (I-STOP) requires real-time reporting and monitoring of controlled substance prescriptions to prevent abuse and diversion. California's Controlled Substance Utilization Review and Evaluation System (CURES) serves a similar purpose, providing a database to track and manage prescriptions for controlled substances.

Electronic prescriptions (e-prescriptions) are increasingly common, and states have different guidelines on their use. While federal law under the DEA permits e-prescriptions for controlled substances, states like Maine and New York mandate the use of e-prescriptions for all medications, barring a few exceptions. Familiarizing yourself with these e-prescribing requirements ensures compliance and smooth workflow in processing prescriptions.

Compounding medications—preparing customized medication doses or forms—also falls under state-specific regulations. States like Texas and California have stringent guidelines for both sterile and non-sterile compounding, ensuring that compounded medications meet safety and quality standards. Adhering to these guidelines is crucial for maintaining the integrity of the medications and safeguarding patient health.

Pharmacy Technician Ratios

Many states regulate the ratio of pharmacy technicians to pharmacists, determining how many technicians can work under the supervision of a single pharmacist. These ratios are designed to ensure adequate oversight and maintain high standards of patient care.

For example, North Carolina allows a maximum of two pharmacy technicians per pharmacist, unless additional technicians are approved by the state board based on specific criteria. Florida permits up to four pharmacy technicians per pharmacist in community pharmacies, while in institutional settings, the ratio can be higher with state board approval.

Understanding and adhering to these ratios is essential for legal compliance and effective pharmacy operations. It ensures that pharmacists can adequately supervise and support their technicians, promoting a safe and efficient work environment.

Recordkeeping and Reporting Requirements

Accurate recordkeeping and reporting are fundamental aspects of pharmacy practice, governed by both federal and state regulations. States may have additional requirements for maintaining records related to prescription orders, inventory, and controlled substances.

In states like New Jersey, pharmacies must retain prescription records for at least five years, while in California, the retention period is three years. These records must be readily accessible for audits and inspections by state regulatory authorities.

Reporting requirements can include the mandatory reporting of prescription errors, adverse drug reactions, and theft or loss of controlled substances. For instance, Texas requires pharmacies to report significant losses of controlled substances to the Texas State Board of Pharmacy and the DEA. Staying compliant with these reporting requirements is vital for maintaining pharmacy integrity and public safety.

Patient Counseling and Confidentiality

Patient counseling is a critical component of pharmacy practice, and state regulations often dictate the circumstances under which it must be provided. While federal law requires pharmacists to offer counseling for Medicaid patients, state laws may extend this requirement to all patients receiving new prescriptions.

For example, Oregon mandates that pharmacists offer counseling for every new prescription and any prescription that has changed in dosage, strength, route of administration, or directions for use. This ensures that patients receive essential information about their medications, promoting safe and effective use.

Confidentiality is equally important, with state regulations often reinforcing the protections provided by federal laws such as HIPAA. States may have additional privacy safeguards, such as restrictions on the use of pharmacy data for marketing purposes. Ensuring compliance with these confidentiality requirements protects patient privacy and builds trust in the healthcare system.

Compliance and Inspections

State boards of pharmacy conduct regular inspections of pharmacies to ensure compliance with all applicable laws and regulations. These inspections can be routine or triggered by specific incidents such as complaints or reports of violations.

During an inspection, regulatory authorities may review prescription records, inventory logs, compounding practices, and adherence to safety protocols. They may also assess the pharmacy's physical premises, including storage conditions and security measures for controlled substances.

Preparing for and cooperating with inspections is a critical aspect of maintaining compliance. Ensuring that all records are up-to-date, staff are trained, and procedures are followed helps prevent violations and promotes a culture of accountability and excellence.

In conclusion, understanding state-specific pharmacy regulations is essential for pharmacy technicians. These regulations encompass a wide range of areas, from licensing and certification to prescription processing and patient counseling. By familiarizing yourself with the laws and guidelines in your state, you can ensure compliance, enhance your professional practice, and contribute to the safe and effective delivery of pharmacy services. This knowledge not only prepares you for the PTCE but also equips you with the tools to navigate the complexities of pharmacy practice with confidence and expertise.

ETHICS AND PRIVACY IN PHARMACY PRACTICE

In the realm of pharmacy practice, ethics and privacy stand as pillars of professional conduct, ensuring that patient care is delivered with integrity and respect. These principles are not mere guidelines but essential components of your role as a pharmacy technician. Adhering to ethical standards and maintaining patient privacy fosters trust, promotes safe and effective care, and upholds the dignity of those you serve.

Understanding Ethical Principles

Ethics in pharmacy practice revolves around several key principles that guide decision-making and professional behavior. These principles include beneficence, nonmaleficence, autonomy, justice, and fidelity.

- **Beneficence** is the commitment to act in the best interest of the patient. As a pharmacy technician, this means ensuring that the medications dispensed are appropriate for the patient's condition and that you provide accurate information to support their health and well-being.
- **Nonmaleficence** is the obligation to do no harm. This principle underlies every action you take, from accurately dispensing medications to double-checking dosages and preventing medication errors. Your diligence helps safeguard patients from potential harm.
- **Autonomy** respects the patient's right to make informed decisions about their own health care. This involves providing patients with comprehensive information about their medications, including benefits, risks, and alternatives, empowering them to make choices that align with their values and preferences.
- **Justice** entails fairness in the distribution of health resources and ensuring that all patients receive equitable care. This principle requires you to treat every patient with the same level of care and respect, regardless of their background or circumstances.
- **Fidelity** is the duty to keep promises and maintain trust. In pharmacy practice, this means honoring the confidentiality of patient information, being reliable in your professional responsibilities, and fostering a trustworthy relationship with patients and colleagues.

Confidentiality and Privacy

Patient confidentiality is a cornerstone of pharmacy ethics, reinforced by laws such as the Health Insurance Portability and Accountability Act (HIPAA). Maintaining confidentiality means safeguarding all personal and health information shared by patients, ensuring it is used only for its intended purposes and disclosed only to authorized individuals.

In your role, you will handle sensitive information daily. This includes patients' medical histories, medication records, and personal details. Protecting this information requires vigilance and adherence to privacy protocols. Here are some key practices:

1. **Secure Storage:** Ensure that all patient records, whether electronic or paper-based, are stored securely. Electronic records should be protected with strong passwords, encryption, and access controls. Physical records should be kept in locked cabinets accessible only to authorized personnel.

2. **Discreet Communication:** When discussing patient information, ensure conversations are held in private settings where unauthorized individuals cannot overhear. This applies to in-person discussions, phone calls, and even digital communications.

3. **Minimal Disclosure:** Share only the necessary information required to fulfill your professional duties. For example, when transferring a prescription to another pharmacy, provide only the details relevant to the prescription, not the patient's entire medical history.

4. **Training and Awareness:** Regularly participate in training sessions on privacy practices and stay updated on changes in privacy laws. Awareness of potential breaches and how to prevent them is crucial for maintaining confidentiality.

Ethical Dilemmas and Decision-Making

Ethical dilemmas are situations where there may be conflicting values or principles at play, making it challenging to determine the right course of action. In pharmacy practice, you may encounter scenarios where ethical decision-making is required. Here's how to navigate such dilemmas:

1. **Identify the Dilemma:** Clearly define the ethical issue at hand. This involves recognizing the conflicting principles or values and understanding the potential impact on the patient and other stakeholders.

2. **Gather Information:** Collect all relevant facts, including patient history, medication details, and any legal or institutional guidelines. Comprehensive information provides a solid foundation for decision-making.

3. **Evaluate Options:** Consider the possible courses of action and their consequences. Reflect on how each option aligns with ethical principles such as beneficence, nonmaleficence, autonomy, justice, and fidelity.

4. **Consult:** Seek input from colleagues, supervisors, or ethics committees if needed. Collaborative discussion can provide new perspectives and support more balanced decision-making.

5. **Make a Decision:** Choose the course of action that best aligns with ethical principles and the patient's best interests. Ensure that your decision is well-documented and communicated to all relevant parties.

6. **Reflect and Learn:** After resolving the dilemma, reflect on the process and the outcome. Consider what went well and what could be improved for future situations. Continuous learning from ethical experiences strengthens your professional practice.

Respecting Cultural and Individual Differences

Ethical pharmacy practice also involves respecting the diverse cultural and individual differences among patients. This means being sensitive to variations in beliefs, values, and practices that may influence patients' healthcare decisions and interactions.

1. **Cultural Competence:** Develop an understanding of different cultural backgrounds and how they may affect health behaviors and expectations. This knowledge helps you provide culturally sensitive care that respects patients' beliefs and traditions.

2. **Effective Communication:** Use clear, respectful language when discussing medications and health information. Avoid jargon and ensure that patients understand the information provided. Consider language barriers and use interpreters or translation services when necessary.

3. **Personalized Care:** Recognize that each patient is unique. Tailor your interactions to meet individual needs and preferences, showing empathy and respect for their personal health journey.

Promoting Ethical Practices in the Workplace

Creating an ethical work environment involves more than individual actions; it requires a collective commitment to upholding ethical standards and fostering a culture of integrity. Here are some strategies to promote ethics in the workplace:

1. **Lead by Example:** Model ethical behavior in all your professional interactions. Your actions set a standard for colleagues and contribute to a culture of accountability and respect.

2. **Encourage Open Dialogue:** Create an environment where ethical concerns can be openly discussed without fear of retribution. Encourage colleagues to speak up about potential ethical issues and support transparent, constructive conversations.

3. **Implement Policies:** Ensure that your workplace has clear, accessible policies on ethics and privacy. Regularly review and update these policies to reflect current laws and best practices.

4. **Provide Training:** Offer ongoing education on ethical practices and privacy laws. Training sessions can reinforce the importance of ethics and provide practical guidance on handling ethical dilemmas.

5. **Recognize Ethical Behavior:** Acknowledge and reward ethical behavior in the workplace. Positive reinforcement encourages continued adherence to ethical standards and highlights the value placed on integrity.

In conclusion, ethics and privacy are fundamental to pharmacy practice, shaping every interaction and decision you make as a pharmacy technician. By adhering to ethical principles, maintaining patient confidentiality, navigating ethical dilemmas thoughtfully, and respecting cultural differences, you contribute to a trustworthy and effective healthcare environment. Promoting ethical practices within your workplace further enhances the quality of care provided to patients. Your commitment to these principles not only prepares you for the PTCE but also establishes a strong foundation for a successful and honorable career in pharmacy.

4. APPLIED PHARMACY PRACTICES

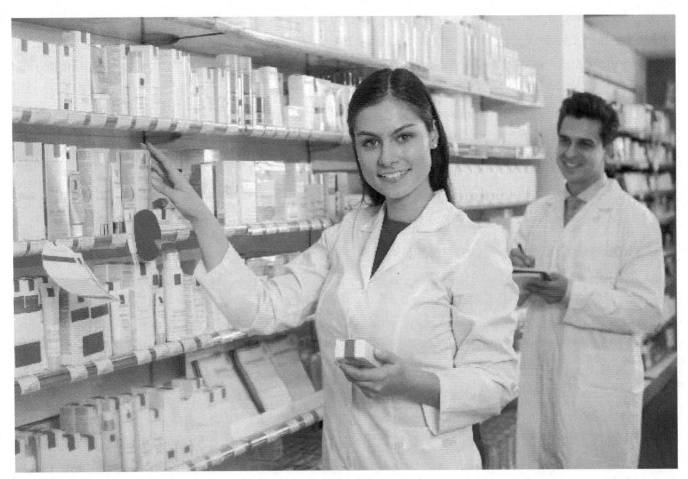

Stepping into the world of applied pharmacy practices means moving beyond theoretical knowledge to the hands-on skills and procedures that define daily operations in a pharmacy. This chapter will immerse you in the practical aspects of pharmacy work, from compounding medications to implementing safety standards and ensuring quality control.

Imagine preparing a sterile compound, carefully measuring and mixing ingredients in a controlled environment, or crafting a personalized medication for a patient with specific needs. These tasks require precision, attention to detail, and a thorough understanding of protocols. In this chapter, you'll learn the essentials of both sterile and non-sterile compounding, gaining insights into the meticulous processes that safeguard patient health.

We'll also explore the critical practices that ensure safety and quality in pharmaceutical services. Whether it's adhering to stringent guidelines to prevent contamination or conducting thorough checks to guarantee the accuracy of prescriptions, these practices are the bedrock of effective pharmacy operations.

By mastering these applied skills, you'll be well-equipped to handle the dynamic and complex nature of pharmacy practice, providing high-quality care and contributing to the overall health and well-being of your patients. Let's delve into the practical side of pharmacy and discover the techniques that turn knowledge into effective action.

Sterile compounding is a critical aspect of pharmacy practice, where precision, cleanliness, and adherence to protocols are paramount. This specialized area involves preparing medications in a sterile environment to prevent contamination and ensure patient safety, often for intravenous use, injections, or ophthalmic preparations. Understanding the basics of sterile compounding equips you with the knowledge to perform these tasks effectively, contributing to high-quality patient care.

The Importance of Sterile Compounding

Sterile compounding is essential for producing medications that must be free from contaminants, including microorganisms, particles, and pyrogens. These preparations are often administered directly into the bloodstream, body tissues, or eyes, where contamination can lead to severe infections or other complications. The standards and practices in sterile compounding are designed to minimize these risks, ensuring that medications are safe and effective.

The Compounding Environment

The environment in which sterile compounding takes place is tightly controlled to maintain sterility. This area is known as the cleanroom or compounding aseptic isolator (CAI), designed to meet strict air quality standards as outlined by USP <797>, the United States Pharmacopeia chapter governing sterile compounding practices.

- **Cleanroom Setup:** A cleanroom typically consists of an anteroom and a buffer area. The anteroom serves as a transition space where personnel can perform hand hygiene, don personal protective equipment (PPE), and minimize the introduction of contaminants. The buffer area is where actual compounding takes place, equipped with laminar airflow workbenches (LAFWs) or biological safety cabinets (BSCs) to ensure a continuous flow of filtered air, maintaining a sterile environment.
- **Air Quality:** The air quality in the compounding area is maintained by high-efficiency particulate air (HEPA) filters, which remove 99.97% of particles that are 0.3 microns or larger. Regular monitoring of air quality, including particle counts and microbial sampling, is essential to ensure compliance with USP <797> standards.

Personal Protective Equipment (PPE)

Proper attire is crucial to prevent contamination in the compounding environment. The PPE required for sterile compounding typically includes:

- **Gowns:** Sterile, lint-free gowns that cover the body to prevent shedding of skin particles and other contaminants.
- **Gloves:** Sterile gloves that are regularly sanitized with isopropyl alcohol to maintain sterility during the compounding process.
- **Face Masks and Goggles:** To protect against respiratory droplets and other contaminants.
- **Hair and Shoe Covers:** To prevent the introduction of hair and other particles into the sterile environment.

Hand Hygiene and Aseptic Technique

Hand hygiene is the first line of defense against contamination. Proper handwashing involves scrubbing hands and forearms with an antimicrobial soap for at least 30 seconds, followed by thorough rinsing and drying with a sterile towel. After donning gloves, hands should be sanitized regularly with 70% isopropyl alcohol.

Aseptic technique refers to the methods used to prevent contamination during the compounding process. Key aspects of aseptic technique include:

- **Proper Handling of Materials:** Only bring necessary items into the sterile field, and disinfect them with 70% isopropyl alcohol before use.
- **Maintaining Sterile Zones:** Work within the designated sterile area, typically the LAFW or BSC, and avoid unnecessary movements that could disturb the airflow.
- **Minimizing Touch Contamination:** Avoid touching critical sites, such as the tips of syringes and needles, with non-sterile surfaces.

Compounding Process

The actual process of sterile compounding involves several precise steps, each requiring careful attention to detail:

- **Preparation:** Gather all necessary materials, including medications, diluents, syringes, needles, and other supplies. Verify that all items are within their expiration dates and have been inspected for integrity.
- **Labeling:** Ensure that each component is correctly labeled, including lot numbers and expiration dates, to maintain traceability and accountability.
- **Compounding:** Follow the specific formula and procedure for the medication being compounded. This may involve reconstituting powdered medications, diluting concentrated solutions, or combining multiple ingredients. Use aseptic technique throughout to prevent contamination.
- **Verification:** Have a pharmacist or another qualified professional verify the accuracy of the compounded preparation, including the correct ingredients, concentrations, and volumes.

Quality Control and Assurance

Ensuring the quality and sterility of compounded medications involves several layers of quality control and assurance:

- **Environmental Monitoring:** Regular monitoring of the compounding environment for particulate and microbial contamination. This includes air and surface sampling, which should be documented and reviewed regularly.
- **Process Validation:** Routine validation of compounding processes to ensure they consistently produce sterile preparations. This may involve media fill tests, where a growth medium is used in place of the actual medication to test for contamination.
- **End-Product Testing:** Testing of the final compounded product for sterility, potency, and the absence of pyrogens. This is particularly important for high-risk or batch-compounded preparations.

Documentation and Record-Keeping

Accurate documentation is critical for ensuring traceability, accountability, and compliance with regulatory standards. Essential records in sterile compounding include:

- **Compounding Logs:** Detailed records of each compounded preparation, including ingredients, lot numbers, quantities, and procedures followed.
- **Quality Control Logs:** Documentation of environmental monitoring results, process validation outcomes, and end-product testing.
- **Personnel Training Records:** Evidence of training and competency assessments for all personnel involved in sterile compounding.

Regulatory Compliance

Compliance with USP <797> is mandatory for all pharmacies engaged in sterile compounding. This standard outlines the requirements for facilities, equipment, personnel, and procedures to ensure the safety and efficacy of compounded sterile preparations. Additionally, state boards of pharmacy and other regulatory bodies may have specific requirements that must be adhered to.

Regular inspections and audits by regulatory authorities help ensure compliance and identify areas for improvement. Staying informed about updates to regulations and best practices is essential for maintaining high standards of quality and safety.

Sterile compounding is a highly specialized and regulated area of pharmacy practice that demands meticulous attention to detail, strict adherence to protocols, and a deep understanding of aseptic techniques. As a pharmacy technician, mastering the basics of sterile compounding equips you with the skills and knowledge to contribute to the safe and effective preparation of medications, ultimately enhancing patient care and outcomes.

By maintaining a clean and controlled environment, using proper personal protective equipment, following aseptic techniques, and adhering to quality control measures, you ensure that every compounded medication meets the highest standards of sterility and quality. This commitment to excellence not only fulfills regulatory requirements but also fosters trust and confidence in the healthcare system.

NON-STERILE COMPOUNDING TECHNIQUES

Non-sterile compounding is a vital aspect of pharmacy practice, allowing for the customization of medications to meet the specific needs of patients. This process involves the preparation of medications in various forms, such as creams, ointments, capsules, and solutions, which do not require a sterile environment but must still adhere to strict standards to ensure safety, efficacy, and quality.

The Importance of Non-Sterile Compounding

Non-sterile compounding provides essential services, particularly for patients who need medications that are not commercially available, require a specific dosage, or have allergies to certain excipients. It also allows for the creation of pediatric dosages, flavoring of medications to improve palatability, and the formulation of medications for veterinary use.

Facilities and Equipment

The environment where non-sterile compounding takes place must be clean, organized, and equipped with the necessary tools to ensure precision and safety. While it does not require the same stringent air quality controls as sterile compounding, maintaining a clean and controlled workspace is essential.

- **Compounding Area:** Designate a specific area within the pharmacy for non-sterile compounding. This area should be free from distractions and contamination sources, with surfaces that are easy to clean and disinfect.
- **Equipment:** Essential equipment includes balances (both electronic and torsion), mortar and pestle, spatulas, graduated cylinders, beakers, hot plates, and mixing devices. All equipment must be calibrated regularly and cleaned thoroughly before and after use to prevent cross-contamination.

Personal Protective Equipment (PPE)

While the PPE requirements for non-sterile compounding are less stringent than for sterile compounding, they are still crucial for protecting both the compounder and the medication from contamination.

- **Gloves:** Always wear disposable gloves to prevent contamination and protect your hands from potentially hazardous substances.
- **Face Masks:** Use face masks when working with powders or other materials that may become airborne.
- **Aprons and Lab Coats:** Wear clean aprons or lab coats to protect your clothing and minimize the risk of introducing contaminants into the compounding area.

Compounding Techniques

The specific techniques used in non-sterile compounding depend on the type of medication being prepared. Here, we explore some of the most common methods.

1. Triturating

Triturating involves grinding a substance to a fine powder. This process is essential for creating uniform particle sizes, which ensures consistent dosing and mixing. A mortar and pestle are typically used for this technique.

- **Procedure:** Place the substance in the mortar and use the pestle to grind it in a circular motion until the desired fineness is achieved. Apply even pressure and continue grinding until no coarse particles remain.

2. Geometric Dilution

Geometric dilution is a method used to evenly distribute a small amount of potent drug throughout a large quantity of diluent. This technique is crucial for ensuring uniform potency in compounded medications.

- **Procedure:** Begin by mixing the potent drug with an equal amount of diluent. Thoroughly triturate the mixture. Add an equal amount of diluent to the mixture and triturate again. Repeat this process until all the diluent has been incorporated, ensuring even distribution of the drug.

3. Levigating

Levigating involves reducing the particle size of a solid by triturating it with a small amount of liquid, known as the levigating agent. This technique is commonly used when incorporating solids into ointments or creams.

- **Procedure:** Place the solid in the mortar and add a small amount of levigating agent, such as mineral oil or glycerin. Use the pestle to triturate the mixture, creating a smooth, uniform paste. This paste can then be incorporated into the base.

4. Spatulation

Spatulation involves mixing ingredients using a spatula on an ointment slab or tile. This technique is suitable for blending powders and semi-solids without creating significant air entrapment.

- **Procedure:** Place the ingredients on the slab and use the spatula to fold and mix them. Continue spatulating until a homogeneous mixture is achieved. This method is often used for preparing ointments and creams.

5. Dissolving and Mixing

Dissolving and mixing are fundamental techniques for preparing solutions and suspensions. Solutions are homogeneous mixtures where the solute is completely dissolved in the solvent, while suspensions are heterogeneous mixtures where the solute particles are dispersed but not dissolved.

- **Procedure for Solutions:** Measure the required amount of solvent (e.g., water, alcohol) and place it in a beaker. Gradually add the solute while stirring continuously until it is fully dissolved.
- **Procedure for Suspensions:** Similar to preparing solutions, but ensure that the solid particles are evenly dispersed throughout the liquid by shaking or stirring. Suspending agents may be added to prevent the particles from settling.

Quality Control and Assurance

Ensuring the quality and safety of compounded non-sterile preparations involves several steps:

- **Ingredient Verification:** Verify the identity and purity of all ingredients before use. Check expiration dates and ensure that the ingredients have been stored properly.
- **Labeling:** Properly label all compounded preparations with the drug name, strength, dosage form, expiration date, and any special storage instructions. Include any warnings or instructions necessary for safe use.
- **Documentation:** Maintain comprehensive records of all compounded preparations, including the formula used, the lot numbers of ingredients, the compounding process, and the personnel involved. Documentation is critical for traceability and accountability.
- **Stability and Beyond-Use Dating:** Assign beyond-use dates based on stability data and storage conditions. This ensures that compounded medications remain effective and safe for use within the specified timeframe.

Patient Counseling

Effective patient counseling is essential to ensure that patients understand how to use their compounded medications correctly. Provide clear instructions on dosage, administration, and storage. Discuss any potential side effects or interactions and emphasize the importance of following the prescribed regimen.

Regulatory Compliance

Non-sterile compounding must comply with USP <795>, which outlines the standards for compounding non-sterile preparations. These standards include guidelines on personnel qualifications, facilities, equipment, component selection, stability, packaging, and documentation. Additionally, stay informed about state-specific regulations and any updates to national standards. Regular audits and inspections by regulatory bodies help ensure compliance and identify areas for improvement.

Non-sterile compounding is a crucial aspect of pharmacy practice that requires precision, attention to detail, and adherence to established protocols. By mastering the techniques of triturating, geometric dilution, levigating, spatulation, and dissolving and mixing, you can prepare a wide range of customized medications to meet the unique needs of patients.

Ensuring quality control, proper labeling, thorough documentation, and patient counseling are all essential components of the compounding process. Adhering to regulatory standards and maintaining a commitment to continuous improvement ensures that non-sterile compounded medications are safe, effective, and of the highest quality.

As a pharmacy technician, your role in non-sterile compounding is vital to providing personalized patient care and enhancing therapeutic outcomes. This knowledge not only prepares you for the practical challenges of compounding but also underscores the importance of precision and professionalism in every aspect of your work.

IMPLEMENTING SAFETY STANDARDS IN MEDICINE HANDLING

Implementing safety standards in medicine handling is essential to ensure patient safety and the integrity of the medications dispensed. As a pharmacy technician, your role in upholding these standards is critical. Let's explore the key practices and protocols that form the foundation of safe medicine handling, from receiving and storing medications to dispensing and disposing of them properly.

Receiving and Inspecting Medications

The process of medicine handling begins with the receipt of medications from suppliers. This initial step is crucial for ensuring that all products meet quality and safety standards before they enter the pharmacy inventory.

- **Verification:** Upon receiving a shipment, verify that the quantities and products match the purchase order. Check the labels, lot numbers, and expiration dates to ensure accuracy. Inspect the packaging for any signs of damage or tampering.
- **Condition Check:** Assess the physical condition of the medications. Look for discoloration, unusual odors, or any signs of contamination. Any discrepancies or concerns should be reported to the supplier immediately, and the affected products should be quarantined until resolved.

Proper Storage Conditions

Once medications have been received and verified, proper storage is essential to maintain their efficacy and safety. Different medications require specific storage conditions, which must be adhered to rigorously.

- **Temperature Control:** Medications must be stored at appropriate temperatures as indicated by the manufacturer. For instance, some medications need refrigeration, while others should be kept at room temperature. Use calibrated thermometers to monitor storage areas regularly, and maintain temperature logs for record-keeping.
- **Humidity Control:** Excess moisture can degrade medications, so it's essential to control humidity levels in storage areas. Dehumidifiers and climate control systems can help maintain optimal conditions.
- **Organization:** Arrange medications in a systematic manner, using a first-in, first-out (FIFO) system to ensure that older stock is used before newer stock. This practice helps prevent expiration and ensures that medications are used within their shelf life.
- **Security:** Store controlled substances in a secure, locked cabinet or safe to prevent theft or unauthorized access. Regularly audit the inventory of controlled substances to ensure accuracy and compliance with regulatory requirements.

Handling Hazardous Medications

Certain medications, such as chemotherapy agents or biohazardous drugs, require special handling due to their potential risks to healthcare workers and patients.

- **Personal Protective Equipment (PPE):** Always wear appropriate PPE, such as gloves, gowns, and face shields, when handling hazardous medications. This protects you from exposure to harmful substances.
- **Designated Areas:** Prepare and handle hazardous medications in designated areas equipped with proper ventilation and containment systems. Use biological safety cabinets (BSCs) or compounding aseptic containment isolators (CACIs) to prevent contamination and exposure.
- **Spill Kits:** Keep spill kits readily available in areas where hazardous medications are handled. These kits should include absorbent materials, neutralizing agents, and disposal bags to manage spills safely and effectively.

Safe Dispensing Practices

Dispensing medications accurately and safely is a core responsibility of pharmacy technicians. This process involves multiple checks and balances to minimize the risk of errors.

- **Prescription Verification:** Carefully review each prescription for accuracy, including the patient's name, medication, dosage, route of administration, and instructions. Verify that the prescription is legible and complete. If there are any uncertainties, consult with the pharmacist or contact the prescriber for clarification.
- **Medication Preparation:** Use precise measuring tools and techniques to prepare the correct dosage. For liquid medications, use calibrated syringes or measuring cups. For solid medications, use counting trays and pill counters to ensure accuracy.

- **Labeling:** Properly label each medication container with the patient's name, medication name, dosage, instructions, and any necessary warnings. Double-check the label against the original prescription to ensure all information is correct.
- **Counseling:** Although counseling is typically the pharmacist's responsibility, as a pharmacy technician, you can support this process by preparing the medication information leaflets and highlighting key points for the pharmacist to discuss with the patient.

Preventing Medication Errors

Medication errors can have serious consequences, so implementing strategies to prevent them is vital.

- **Standard Operating Procedures (SOPs):** Adhere to SOPs for all tasks, from prescription verification to dispensing. SOPs provide a structured approach to pharmacy operations, reducing variability and minimizing the risk of errors.
- **Barcoding:** Utilize barcode technology to verify medications during dispensing. Scanning the barcode ensures that the correct medication and dosage are selected, matching the prescription and reducing the likelihood of human error.
- **Double-Check System:** Implement a double-check system where another pharmacy technician or pharmacist reviews the prepared medication before it is dispensed. This additional layer of verification helps catch potential errors.
- **Continuing Education:** Stay informed about best practices, new medications, and emerging safety standards through continuing education and training. Regular updates help you maintain competency and stay current with industry developments.

Disposing of Medications Safely

Proper disposal of medications is essential to prevent environmental contamination and misuse. Follow guidelines for disposing of expired, unused, or contaminated medications.

- **Take-Back Programs:** Participate in or promote medication take-back programs that allow patients to return unused medications to the pharmacy for safe disposal. These programs help prevent misuse and protect the environment.
- **Hazardous Waste Disposal:** Dispose of hazardous medications according to local, state, and federal regulations. Use designated containers for hazardous waste, and ensure that they are handled by licensed disposal companies.
- **Controlled Substances:** Follow DEA regulations for the disposal of controlled substances. This may involve using specific disposal methods, such as incineration or chemical deactivation, to ensure that these substances are rendered non-retrievable.

Documentation and Record-Keeping

Maintaining accurate records is crucial for ensuring accountability and traceability in medicine handling.

- **Inventory Logs:** Keep detailed logs of all medications received, dispensed, and disposed of. Regularly reconcile inventory records with physical counts to identify and address discrepancies promptly.

- **Temperature and Humidity Logs:** Document temperature and humidity readings for storage areas to demonstrate compliance with storage requirements.
- **Training Records:** Maintain records of training and competency assessments for all staff involved in medication handling. This documentation supports ongoing education and ensures that personnel are qualified to perform their duties safely.

Continuous Improvement

Implementing safety standards in medicine handling is an ongoing process that requires regular review and improvement.

- **Audits and Inspections:** Conduct regular internal audits and inspections to assess compliance with safety standards and identify areas for improvement. Address any findings promptly and implement corrective actions.
- **Feedback Mechanisms:** Encourage staff to provide feedback on current practices and suggest improvements. Creating an open environment where concerns can be raised and addressed helps foster a culture of safety.
- **Root Cause Analysis:** When errors or incidents occur, perform a root cause analysis to understand the underlying factors and develop strategies to prevent recurrence. This proactive approach enhances safety and quality.

Implementing safety standards in medicine handling is fundamental to ensuring patient safety and maintaining the integrity of the pharmacy profession. By adhering to protocols for receiving, storing, dispensing, and disposing of medications, you play a crucial role in minimizing risks and ensuring that medications are handled correctly.

Through diligent practice, continuous education, and a commitment to excellence, you contribute to a safe and effective pharmacy environment. Your attention to detail and adherence to safety standards not only protect patients but also uphold the trust and confidence placed in the pharmacy by the community. This commitment to safety is a cornerstone of your professional practice and a vital component of providing high-quality healthcare.

PRACTICES FOR ENSURING QUALITY IN PHARMACEUTICAL SERVICES

Ensuring quality in pharmaceutical services is a multifaceted endeavor that encompasses a range of practices aimed at maintaining the highest standards of safety, efficacy, and patient care. As a pharmacy technician, your role in this process is vital. From compounding and dispensing medications to patient interactions and adherence to regulatory guidelines, every aspect of your work contributes to the overall quality of pharmaceutical services. Let's delve into the key practices that uphold these standards.

Accurate Prescription Processing

The foundation of quality pharmaceutical services lies in the accurate processing of prescriptions. This begins with thorough verification to ensure that all prescription details are correct and complete.

- **Verification:** Carefully check the patient's name, date of birth, medication name, dosage, route of administration, and instructions. Verify the prescriber's information and ensure the prescription is legible and valid. Any uncertainties should prompt a consultation with the pharmacist or a call to the prescriber for clarification.
- **Documentation:** Maintain detailed records of each prescription processed, including any modifications or clarifications. Accurate documentation ensures traceability and accountability, facilitating quality control and audits.

Adherence to Compounding Standards

When compounding medications, adherence to established standards ensures that the preparations are safe, effective, and of high quality. This involves precise measurements, proper techniques, and rigorous quality checks.

- **Formulation and Ingredients:** Use validated formulas and high-quality ingredients. Verify the identity and purity of all components before use, and ensure they are within their expiration dates.
- **Compounding Environment:** Maintain a clean and organized compounding area. For sterile compounding, follow USP <797> guidelines to ensure a contaminant-free environment. For non-sterile compounding, adhere to USP <795> standards.
- **Quality Control:** Implement checks at each stage of the compounding process. This includes verifying calculations, inspecting the final product for consistency and appearance, and performing potency tests when necessary.

Stringent Labeling and Packaging

Proper labeling and packaging are critical for ensuring that patients receive the correct medications with the appropriate instructions and warnings.

- **Labeling:** Labels should clearly display the patient's name, medication name, dosage, administration route, and any special instructions or warnings. Double-check labels against the original prescription to ensure accuracy.
- **Packaging:** Use appropriate packaging to protect the medication's integrity. For example, child-resistant containers help prevent accidental ingestion, while amber bottles protect light-sensitive medications. Ensure that packaging is tamper-evident and provides adequate protection during storage and transport.

Patient Safety and Error Prevention

Minimizing the risk of medication errors is a cornerstone of quality pharmaceutical services. Implementing systems and practices that promote accuracy and safety is essential.

- **Standard Operating Procedures (SOPs):** Develop and adhere to SOPs for all pharmacy tasks. SOPs provide a consistent framework for operations, reducing variability and the likelihood of errors.

- **Double-Check System:** Incorporate a double-check system where another technician or pharmacist reviews the prepared medication before dispensing. This additional verification step helps catch errors and ensures accuracy.
- **Technology Integration:** Utilize technology such as electronic prescribing, barcode scanning, and automated dispensing systems. These tools enhance accuracy and streamline workflow, reducing the potential for human error.

Effective Communication and Counseling

Clear communication with patients and healthcare providers is essential for ensuring the safe and effective use of medications.

- **Patient Counseling:** Provide patients with comprehensive information about their medications, including how to take them, potential side effects, and storage instructions. Encourage questions and ensure that patients understand their treatment regimen.
- **Provider Collaboration:** Maintain open lines of communication with prescribers and other healthcare professionals. Promptly address any questions or concerns about prescriptions, and share relevant patient information to support coordinated care.

Continuous Monitoring and Improvement

Quality assurance in pharmaceutical services is an ongoing process that involves regular monitoring and continuous improvement.

- **Audits and Inspections:** Conduct regular internal audits and inspections to assess compliance with standards and identify areas for improvement. External audits by regulatory bodies also play a crucial role in maintaining quality.
- **Feedback Mechanisms:** Implement systems for collecting feedback from patients and staff. This input can highlight strengths and reveal areas needing improvement, guiding quality enhancement initiatives.
- **Root Cause Analysis:** When errors or incidents occur, perform a root cause analysis to understand the underlying factors and develop strategies to prevent recurrence. This proactive approach promotes a culture of safety and quality.

Training and Professional Development

Ongoing training and professional development are vital for maintaining high standards in pharmaceutical services. Ensuring that all staff members are knowledgeable and skilled supports quality and safety.

- **Initial Training:** Provide comprehensive training for new staff members, covering all aspects of pharmacy operations, including compounding techniques, medication safety, and regulatory compliance.
- **Continuing Education:** Encourage and facilitate continuing education for all staff. Staying current with the latest advancements, guidelines, and best practices ensures that the pharmacy team can provide high-quality care.
- **Competency Assessments:** Regularly assess the competencies of staff members through practical evaluations and knowledge tests. This helps identify areas where additional training or support may be needed.

Regulatory Compliance

Adherence to regulatory standards and guidelines is a fundamental aspect of ensuring quality in pharmaceutical services. Compliance with these standards protects patient safety and supports the pharmacy's credibility and legal standing.

- **USP Standards:** Follow USP guidelines for compounding, labeling, and storage of medications. These standards provide a comprehensive framework for ensuring the quality and safety of pharmaceutical preparations.
- **DEA Regulations:** Comply with DEA regulations for handling controlled substances, including secure storage, accurate recordkeeping, and proper disposal. Regularly review and update practices to align with current regulations.
- **State Board Requirements:** Stay informed about state-specific regulations and ensure that all practices meet the requirements set by the state board of pharmacy. This includes licensing, continuing education, and operational standards.

Patient-Centered Care

At the heart of quality pharmaceutical services is a commitment to patient-centered care. This involves not only providing accurate and safe medications but also ensuring that patients feel supported and informed.

- **Personalized Services:** Tailor services to meet the unique needs of each patient. This may include customizing dosages, offering medication synchronization, or providing special packaging for ease of use.
- **Empathy and Support:** Approach patient interactions with empathy and a supportive attitude. Listen to patients' concerns, provide reassurance, and offer assistance in managing their medications and overall health.

Ensuring quality in pharmaceutical services is a multifaceted responsibility that encompasses accurate prescription processing, adherence to compounding standards, stringent labeling and packaging, error prevention, effective communication, continuous monitoring, training, regulatory compliance, and patient-centered care. Each of these elements plays a crucial role in maintaining the highest standards of safety, efficacy, and patient satisfaction.

As a pharmacy technician, your dedication to these practices not only upholds the integrity of the pharmacy profession but also significantly impacts the health and well-being of the patients you serve. By embracing a commitment to excellence and continuous improvement, you contribute to a culture of quality that defines exceptional pharmaceutical care. This holistic approach ensures that every aspect of your work meets the highest standards, fostering trust and confidence in the services provided.

5. PHARMACY OPERATIONS

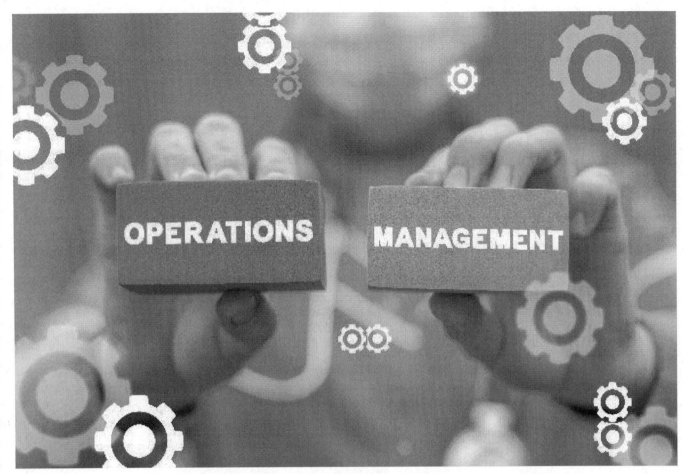

Navigating the intricate world of pharmacy operations is akin to orchestrating a finely tuned symphony. Every aspect, from inventory management to workflow optimization, plays a critical role in ensuring the seamless delivery of healthcare services. This chapter delves into the heart of pharmacy operations, shedding light on the essential components that keep a pharmacy running smoothly and efficiently.

Imagine the daily rhythm of a bustling pharmacy: patients arriving with prescriptions, the meticulous preparation of medications, and the constant vigilance required to maintain accurate records and inventory. Each task, no matter how small, contributes to the overall harmony of the pharmacy. In this chapter, we'll explore the systems and strategies that underpin effective pharmacy operations.

We'll start with an in-depth look at pharmacy information systems, the digital backbone that supports all facets of pharmacy work. From there, we'll examine techniques for order entry and processing, ensuring accuracy and efficiency in every transaction. Inventory management will also be a focal point, highlighting methods to maintain optimal stock levels and reduce waste.

By understanding these operational foundations, you'll be equipped to contribute to a pharmacy environment that is not only efficient but also responsive to the needs of patients and healthcare providers. Let's embark on this journey to master the complexities of pharmacy operations and ensure the highest standards of service and care.

Pharmacy Information Systems (PIS) are the technological backbone of modern pharmacy operations, transforming the way pharmacists and pharmacy technicians manage prescriptions, patient information, inventory, and regulatory compliance. Understanding the role and operations of these systems is essential for optimizing efficiency, accuracy, and patient care within a pharmacy.

The Role of Pharmacy Information Systems

Pharmacy Information Systems are designed to streamline various pharmacy processes, integrating multiple functions into a cohesive platform. They provide a comprehensive framework that supports medication management, patient safety, regulatory compliance, and operational efficiency. Let's explore how these systems impact key areas of pharmacy practice.

1. Medication Management

One of the primary functions of a PIS is to manage the medication-use process. This includes prescription entry, medication dispensing, and monitoring of drug therapies.

- **Prescription Entry:** PIS allows for the electronic entry of prescriptions, reducing the risk of errors associated with handwritten prescriptions. Electronic prescriptions can be transmitted directly from healthcare providers to the pharmacy, ensuring clarity and accuracy. The system verifies the prescription details, including dosage, quantity, and instructions, and checks for potential drug interactions or allergies.

- **Medication Dispensing:** Once a prescription is entered, the PIS facilitates the dispensing process by generating labels, providing compounding instructions, and tracking the medication through each step of preparation. Automated dispensing systems, integrated with the PIS, further enhance accuracy by precisely measuring and dispensing medications.

- **Drug Monitoring:** PIS includes tools for monitoring drug therapies, such as drug utilization reviews (DURs) and medication therapy management (MTM). These tools help identify potential issues, such as therapeutic duplications, contraindications, and non-adherence, allowing pharmacists to intervene and optimize patient outcomes.

2. Patient Safety

Enhancing patient safety is a critical goal of any PIS. These systems incorporate various features to minimize the risk of medication errors and ensure safe medication use.

- **Clinical Decision Support:** PIS provides clinical decision support tools that alert pharmacists and technicians to potential drug interactions, allergies, and contraindications. These alerts prompt further review and verification, reducing the likelihood of adverse drug events.

- **Barcoding:** The integration of barcode scanning technology with the PIS ensures that the correct medication is dispensed to the right patient. Each medication is scanned and verified against the prescription details, minimizing errors and enhancing safety.

- **Patient Profiles:** PIS maintains comprehensive patient profiles that include medication histories, allergies, and preferences. Access to this information enables pharmacists to make informed decisions and provide personalized care.

3. Inventory Management

Efficient inventory management is essential for maintaining optimal stock levels, reducing waste, and ensuring that medications are available when needed. PIS plays a crucial role in this aspect by automating and streamlining inventory processes.

- **Automated Inventory Tracking:** PIS tracks inventory levels in real-time, updating stock counts as medications are dispensed. This real-time tracking helps prevent stockouts and overstock situations, ensuring that the pharmacy maintains an optimal inventory balance.

- **Order Management:** PIS generates purchase orders based on predefined reorder points and usage patterns. Automated ordering reduces the administrative burden on staff and ensures timely replenishment of stock. The system also tracks the status of orders, from placement to receipt, providing complete visibility into the inventory supply chain.

- **Expiration Date Monitoring:** PIS monitors the expiration dates of medications in inventory, alerting staff to upcoming expirations. This proactive approach allows for timely removal or return of expired medications, reducing waste and ensuring that only safe, effective medications are dispensed.

4. Regulatory Compliance

Compliance with regulatory requirements is a critical aspect of pharmacy operations. PIS supports compliance efforts by maintaining accurate records, facilitating reporting, and ensuring adherence to laws and guidelines.

- **Record-Keeping:** PIS maintains detailed records of all pharmacy transactions, including prescription entries, dispensed medications, inventory adjustments, and patient interactions. These records are essential for audits, inspections, and compliance with regulatory agencies such as the DEA and FDA.

- **Reporting:** PIS generates various reports required for regulatory compliance, such as controlled substance inventories, dispensing logs, and adverse event reports. Automated reporting features ensure that required documentation is complete, accurate, and submitted on time.

- **Regulatory Updates:** PIS systems are regularly updated to reflect changes in regulatory requirements and guidelines. This ensures that the pharmacy remains compliant with the latest laws and standards, reducing the risk of non-compliance and associated penalties.

5. Operational Efficiency

PIS enhances the overall efficiency of pharmacy operations by automating routine tasks, reducing manual workload, and improving workflow.

- **Task Automation:** Routine tasks such as prescription entry, labeling, and inventory management are automated, freeing up staff time for more critical activities. Automation reduces the risk of human error and increases overall productivity.

- **Workflow Optimization:** PIS provides tools for optimizing workflow, such as task prioritization, resource allocation, and workload balancing. These tools help streamline processes, reduce bottlenecks, and ensure that pharmacy operations run smoothly.

- **Data Integration:** PIS integrates data from various sources, including electronic health records (EHRs), laboratory systems, and insurance databases. This integration provides a comprehensive view of patient information, enabling more informed decision-making and coordinated care.

Implementing and Maintaining Pharmacy Information Systems

Implementing a PIS requires careful planning, training, and ongoing maintenance to ensure its effectiveness and longevity.

- **Planning and Implementation:** Selecting and implementing a PIS involves assessing the pharmacy's needs, evaluating system features, and planning for integration with existing systems. A thorough implementation plan includes timelines, resource allocation, and training schedules.
- **Training:** Comprehensive training is essential for ensuring that all staff members are proficient in using the PIS. Training should cover system navigation, data entry, report generation, and troubleshooting. Ongoing training and refreshers help keep staff updated on system features and best practices.
- **Maintenance and Support:** Regular maintenance and support are critical for ensuring the smooth operation of the PIS. This includes software updates, hardware maintenance, and technical support. Establishing a relationship with the PIS vendor for ongoing support and troubleshooting is essential.

Pharmacy Information Systems are integral to modern pharmacy operations, providing a robust framework for medication management, patient safety, inventory control, regulatory compliance, and operational efficiency. As a pharmacy technician, understanding the role and operations of PIS empowers you to leverage technology effectively, enhancing the quality of care provided to patients. By integrating these systems into daily practices, pharmacies can achieve greater accuracy, efficiency, and safety in their operations. Continuous learning and adaptation to new technologies and features ensure that pharmacy staff remain proficient and that the PIS continues to meet the evolving needs of the pharmacy and its patients. This commitment to excellence in technology and practice underscores the critical role of PIS in delivering high-quality pharmaceutical services.

EFFICIENT TECHNIQUES IN ORDER ENTRY AND PROCESSING

Efficient order entry and processing are vital components of pharmacy operations, directly impacting the accuracy, speed, and quality of patient care. Streamlining these processes ensures that prescriptions are filled correctly and promptly, reducing the potential for errors and enhancing overall efficiency. Here, we explore effective techniques for managing order entry and processing in a pharmacy setting.

Streamlining Prescription Intake

The first step in efficient order entry and processing is optimizing how prescriptions are received and recorded. This involves implementing systems and practices that facilitate smooth and accurate intake of prescriptions from various sources.

- **Electronic Prescriptions (E-Prescribing):** Leveraging electronic prescribing systems reduces the risk of errors associated with handwritten prescriptions. E-prescriptions are transmitted directly from the healthcare provider to the pharmacy's information system, ensuring clarity and accuracy. This not only speeds up the intake process but also facilitates automatic checks for drug interactions and allergies.
- **Standardized Forms:** For prescriptions received in writing or verbally, using standardized intake forms helps ensure all necessary information is captured consistently. These forms should include fields for patient information, medication details, dosage instructions, and prescriber information.
- **Centralized Intake Points:** Designating specific intake points within the pharmacy for receiving prescriptions helps streamline the process. Whether it's a dedicated counter, drop-off box, or online portal, having a clear and organized intake system reduces confusion and bottlenecks.

Accurate Data Entry

Once a prescription is received, entering the data accurately into the pharmacy information system (PIS) is crucial. This step involves several techniques to ensure precision and efficiency.

- **Double-Check Protocols:** Implementing a double-check system where two staff members verify the entered information can significantly reduce errors. This process involves one person entering the data and another reviewing it for accuracy before it is finalized.
- **Use of Templates and Defaults:** Utilizing templates and default settings in the PIS can streamline data entry for common medications and dosage instructions. These pre-configured settings ensure consistency and save time, especially for frequently prescribed medications.
- **Real-Time Data Entry:** Entering prescription information in real-time, as it is received, minimizes the risk of transcription errors and ensures that the data is up-to-date. This practice is particularly important in busy pharmacy environments where delays can lead to mistakes.

Enhancing Workflow Efficiency

Optimizing the workflow for order processing involves structuring tasks and responsibilities to maximize efficiency and minimize delays.

- **Task Segmentation:** Dividing the order processing workflow into distinct tasks—such as data entry, verification, preparation, and dispensing—allows staff to focus on specific responsibilities. This segmentation can enhance productivity and reduce the likelihood of errors.
- **Workflow Automation:** Implementing automation tools within the PIS can streamline various aspects of order processing. For example, automated alerts for drug interactions, automatic label generation, and electronic tracking of order status help maintain a smooth workflow.

- **Queue Management:** Effective queue management systems prioritize and organize prescriptions based on urgency and complexity. This ensures that high-priority orders, such as acute medications, are processed quickly, while routine prescriptions are handled efficiently.

Verification and Quality Control

Ensuring the accuracy and quality of processed orders is essential for maintaining patient safety and trust.

- **Pharmacist Verification:** A crucial step in the order processing workflow is the pharmacist's verification. After the data entry and initial processing, the pharmacist reviews the prescription for accuracy, appropriateness, and potential interactions. This step is vital for catching any discrepancies before the medication is dispensed.
- **Quality Control Checks:** Implementing regular quality control checks throughout the order processing workflow helps identify and address errors early. These checks can include verifying the correct medication, dosage, and patient information at multiple points in the process.
- **Barcode Scanning:** Integrating barcode scanning technology with the PIS enhances accuracy by verifying that the correct medication is selected and dispensed. Scanning the barcode on the medication and matching it with the prescription details reduces the risk of dispensing errors.

Effective Communication and Coordination

Clear communication and coordination among pharmacy staff and with patients are essential for efficient order processing.

- **Internal Communication:** Establishing clear communication channels among pharmacy staff helps coordinate tasks and address any issues that arise during order processing. Regular team meetings and use of communication tools such as intercoms or messaging apps can facilitate effective coordination.
- **Patient Communication:** Keeping patients informed about the status of their prescriptions and providing clear instructions for medication use enhances their experience and compliance. Automated notification systems that send alerts via text or email when prescriptions are ready for pickup can improve efficiency and patient satisfaction.

Continuous Improvement and Training

Ongoing training and continuous improvement initiatives are crucial for maintaining and enhancing order processing efficiency.

- **Staff Training:** Regular training sessions for pharmacy staff on the latest PIS features, order processing protocols, and best practices help maintain high standards of efficiency and accuracy. This training should cover both technical skills and customer service practices.
- **Process Evaluation:** Continuously evaluating and refining order processing workflows based on performance metrics and feedback helps identify areas for improvement. Regularly reviewing error rates, processing times, and patient satisfaction scores can guide process enhancements.

- **Technology Updates:** Keeping the PIS and related technologies updated with the latest software and features ensures that the pharmacy can leverage the most efficient tools available. Regular updates and maintenance help prevent technical issues that can disrupt workflow.

Efficient techniques in order entry and processing are fundamental to the smooth operation of a pharmacy. By optimizing prescription intake, ensuring accurate data entry, enhancing workflow efficiency, implementing robust verification and quality control measures, and fostering effective communication and continuous improvement, pharmacies can deliver high-quality, timely, and accurate services to patients.

As a pharmacy technician, mastering these techniques not only improves your workflow but also enhances the overall efficiency and effectiveness of the pharmacy. This commitment to excellence ensures that patients receive their medications safely and promptly, reinforcing the trust and reliability that are the hallmarks of quality pharmaceutical care. By embracing these best practices, you contribute to a pharmacy environment that prioritizes patient safety, satisfaction, and operational excellence.

ESSENTIAL PHARMACY INVENTORY MANAGEMENT

Effective pharmacy inventory management is crucial for ensuring that medications are available when needed, minimizing waste, and maintaining financial stability. As a pharmacy technician, mastering inventory management practices allows you to contribute to a smoothly operating pharmacy, where patient needs are met promptly and efficiently. Let's explore the essential components of effective inventory management, from procurement and storage to monitoring and disposal.

Procurement and Receiving

The inventory management process begins with procurement—sourcing and ordering the necessary medications and supplies. This step involves careful planning and coordination to ensure that the pharmacy's inventory levels are optimized.

- **Demand Forecasting:** Predicting the demand for medications is a critical aspect of procurement. This involves analyzing historical data, considering seasonal trends, and staying informed about potential changes in prescribing patterns. Effective forecasting helps prevent stockouts and overstock situations.
- **Vendor Relationships:** Establishing strong relationships with reliable suppliers ensures timely and consistent delivery of medications. Regular communication with vendors helps negotiate better terms, manage lead times, and address any issues promptly.
- **Order Placement:** When placing orders, it's essential to use an efficient and accurate system. Many pharmacies utilize automated ordering systems integrated with their Pharmacy Information Systems (PIS), which generate purchase orders based on predefined reorder points and usage patterns. This automation reduces manual errors and streamlines the ordering process.

- **Receiving Shipments:** Upon receiving shipments, carefully inspect all items against the purchase order. Verify that the quantities, lot numbers, and expiration dates match the order. Check for any signs of damage or tampering and report discrepancies to the supplier immediately.

Storage and Organization

Proper storage and organization of inventory are vital for maintaining the quality and integrity of medications. This includes ensuring appropriate environmental conditions and systematic arrangement of stock.

- **Temperature Control:** Medications must be stored at the appropriate temperatures as specified by the manufacturer. This often involves maintaining refrigeration for certain medications and ensuring that the storage area is climate-controlled. Regularly monitor and record temperatures to comply with regulatory standards and ensure the medications remain effective.
- **Humidity Control:** Excess humidity can degrade medications, so it's important to control moisture levels in storage areas. Dehumidifiers and proper ventilation can help maintain an optimal environment.
- **Systematic Arrangement:** Organize medications in a logical and systematic manner. Common practices include alphabetizing by generic name, grouping by therapeutic class, and using the first-in, first-out (FIFO) method to rotate stock. Clearly label all shelves and bins to facilitate easy identification and retrieval.
- **Security:** Secure storage is essential, particularly for controlled substances. These medications should be kept in locked cabinets or safes, with access restricted to authorized personnel. Regular audits and inventory counts help ensure compliance with security protocols.

Inventory Monitoring and Control

Ongoing monitoring and control of inventory levels are crucial for maintaining an efficient pharmacy operation. This involves tracking stock, managing expiration dates, and conducting regular audits.

- **Inventory Tracking:** Use an inventory management system to track stock levels in real-time. These systems provide visibility into current inventory, highlight low stock levels, and trigger reorder alerts. Accurate tracking helps prevent stockouts and overstock situations.
- **Expiration Date Management:** Monitor expiration dates closely and implement a system to identify and remove expired or near-expiration medications. Many pharmacies use color-coded labels or shelf tags to highlight medications nearing their expiration dates, ensuring they are used first.
- **Cycle Counts:** Conduct regular cycle counts—partial inventory counts performed on a rotating basis—to verify inventory accuracy. These counts help identify discrepancies early and allow for timely corrective actions. Full inventory audits should also be conducted periodically to reconcile inventory records with physical counts.

Reducing Waste and Managing Returns

Minimizing waste and managing returns effectively are essential for both financial sustainability and environmental responsibility.

- **Stock Optimization:** Avoid over-ordering by using demand forecasting and inventory tracking data to order the right quantities. Stock optimization techniques, such as just-in-time (JIT) inventory, can help reduce excess stock and associated carrying costs.

- **Managing Returns:** Establish procedures for managing returns from patients and to suppliers. For patient returns, follow regulatory guidelines for handling and disposing of returned medications. For supplier returns, negotiate return policies and credit terms to minimize financial loss.

- **Disposal of Expired and Unusable Medications:** Dispose of expired, damaged, or unusable medications in accordance with local, state, and federal regulations. Use environmentally safe disposal methods, such as incineration or drug take-back programs, to prevent environmental contamination.

Leveraging Technology

Technology plays a significant role in modern pharmacy inventory management, providing tools for automation, data analysis, and process optimization.

- **Inventory Management Software:** Utilize specialized inventory management software integrated with the PIS to automate tracking, ordering, and reporting. These systems enhance accuracy and efficiency by reducing manual tasks and providing real-time insights.

- **Barcode Scanning:** Implement barcode scanning technology to streamline inventory tracking and reduce errors. Scanning barcodes during receiving, dispensing, and audits ensures accurate data entry and inventory counts.

- **Data Analytics:** Leverage data analytics to gain insights into inventory trends, usage patterns, and financial performance. Analyzing data helps identify opportunities for cost savings, process improvements, and better inventory control.

Staff Training and Involvement

Effective inventory management requires the involvement and cooperation of all pharmacy staff. Providing proper training and fostering a collaborative environment are key to success.

- **Training Programs:** Develop comprehensive training programs for new and existing staff, covering inventory management procedures, use of technology, and regulatory compliance. Ongoing training ensures that staff stay current with best practices and new developments.

- **Clear Communication:** Maintain open lines of communication among staff regarding inventory management tasks and responsibilities. Regular team meetings and updates help keep everyone informed and aligned with inventory goals.

- **Empowerment and Accountability:** Empower staff to take ownership of inventory-related tasks and hold them accountable for their responsibilities. Recognize and reward efforts to improve inventory management and reduce waste.

Continuous Improvement

Inventory management is an ongoing process that benefits from continuous evaluation and improvement. Regularly reviewing performance metrics and seeking feedback can drive enhancements.

- **Performance Metrics:** Track key performance indicators (KPIs) such as inventory turnover rate, stockout frequency, and waste reduction. Use these metrics to assess the effectiveness of inventory management practices and identify areas for improvement.
- **Feedback and Adaptation:** Encourage staff to provide feedback on inventory management processes and suggest improvements. Adapting to changing needs and incorporating new ideas helps maintain a dynamic and responsive inventory system.
- **Process Reviews:** Conduct periodic reviews of inventory management processes to ensure they remain effective and aligned with best practices. Adjust procedures as needed to address challenges and optimize performance.

Essential pharmacy inventory management involves a comprehensive approach that encompasses procurement, storage, monitoring, waste reduction, technology utilization, staff training, and continuous improvement. By mastering these elements, pharmacy technicians can ensure that medications are available when needed, maintain high standards of safety and quality, and contribute to the overall efficiency and sustainability of the pharmacy.

Effective inventory management not only supports the day-to-day operations of the pharmacy but also enhances patient care by ensuring that the right medications are available at the right time. This commitment to excellence in inventory management reflects the broader goal of providing reliable, high-quality pharmaceutical services to the community.

OPTIMIZING WORKFLOW IN PHARMACY SETTINGS

Optimizing workflow in pharmacy settings is essential to ensure efficiency, accuracy, and high-quality patient care. A well-structured workflow minimizes errors, reduces wait times, and enhances overall productivity, allowing the pharmacy to operate smoothly even during peak times. Let's explore key strategies and practices for streamlining workflow in a pharmacy setting, from designing an effective layout to leveraging technology and fostering teamwork.

Designing an Effective Layout

The physical layout of the pharmacy plays a significant role in optimizing workflow. A well-designed workspace facilitates smooth movement, minimizes congestion, and ensures that all necessary tools and medications are easily accessible.

- **Zoning:** Divide the pharmacy into functional zones based on different tasks. Common zones include prescription intake, compounding, dispensing, counseling, and storage. Each zone should be equipped with the necessary tools and supplies to perform its specific functions efficiently.
- **Workstations:** Designate specific workstations for key tasks. For instance, have a dedicated area for prescription data entry, another for medication preparation, and separate spaces for pharmacists to verify prescriptions and counsel patients. Ensure that each workstation is ergonomically designed to reduce strain and improve productivity.
- **Flow Paths:** Establish clear and unobstructed flow paths between different zones and workstations. This minimizes unnecessary movement and reduces the risk of collisions and congestion. Use visual cues, such as floor markings or signage, to guide staff and streamline movement.

Task Segmentation and Role Clarity

Clear definition and segmentation of tasks ensure that all team members know their responsibilities and can perform them efficiently.

- **Role Assignment:** Clearly assign roles and responsibilities to each team member based on their skills and expertise. This ensures that tasks are performed by the most qualified individuals, improving accuracy and efficiency. For example, pharmacy technicians can handle prescription intake and data entry, while pharmacists focus on verification and patient counseling.
- **Task Rotation:** Implement task rotation schedules to prevent fatigue and maintain engagement among staff. Rotating tasks ensures that all team members are cross-trained and capable of performing various functions, which enhances flexibility and coverage.
- **Standard Operating Procedures (SOPs):** Develop and adhere to SOPs for all tasks within the pharmacy. SOPs provide a structured framework for operations, ensuring consistency and reducing the likelihood of errors. Regularly review and update SOPs to reflect best practices and new regulatory requirements.

Leveraging Technology

Technology plays a crucial role in optimizing workflow by automating routine tasks, improving accuracy, and enhancing communication.

- **Pharmacy Information Systems (PIS):** Implement a robust PIS to manage all aspects of pharmacy operations, from prescription entry and inventory management to billing and reporting. A well-integrated PIS streamlines processes, reduces manual workload, and provides real-time data for better decision-making.

- **Automated Dispensing Systems:** Utilize automated dispensing systems to accurately count, package, and label medications. These systems reduce the risk of dispensing errors and free up staff time for more critical tasks.
- **Electronic Health Records (EHRs):** Integrate the pharmacy's PIS with EHRs to facilitate seamless communication and data sharing with healthcare providers. This integration ensures that pharmacists have access to comprehensive patient information, enabling better clinical decisions and coordination of care.

Efficient Communication

Effective communication is essential for coordinating tasks, addressing issues promptly, and ensuring smooth workflow.

- **Communication Tools:** Use communication tools such as intercom systems, instant messaging apps, or task management software to facilitate real-time communication among staff. These tools help quickly relay important information and coordinate tasks efficiently.
- **Briefings and Huddles:** Conduct regular briefings or huddles to discuss the day's tasks, address any concerns, and share important updates. These meetings provide an opportunity for team members to align their efforts and ensure everyone is on the same page.
- **Feedback Mechanisms:** Establish feedback mechanisms to encourage open communication and continuous improvement. Encourage staff to share suggestions for workflow enhancements and promptly address any issues that arise.

Managing Workload and Prioritization

Effective workload management and task prioritization are key to maintaining a smooth workflow, especially during busy periods.

- **Task Prioritization:** Implement a system for prioritizing tasks based on urgency and importance. For example, prioritize prescription refills for patients waiting in the pharmacy and urgent medication orders from healthcare providers. Use visual cues, such as color-coded labels or digital dashboards, to indicate priority levels.
- **Queue Management:** Use queue management systems to organize and manage patient flow. These systems can provide estimated wait times, update patients on the status of their prescriptions, and help staff manage their workload more effectively.
- **Capacity Planning:** Regularly assess the pharmacy's capacity and adjust staffing levels accordingly. During peak times, such as flu season or holidays, consider increasing staff or adjusting shifts to ensure adequate coverage.

Training and Continuous Improvement

Ongoing training and a commitment to continuous improvement are essential for maintaining an optimized workflow.

- **Staff Training:** Provide comprehensive training for new hires and ongoing training for existing staff. Training should cover technical skills, use of technology, SOPs, and customer service practices. Well-trained staff are more efficient and better equipped to handle their tasks.

- **Process Evaluation:** Continuously evaluate and refine workflow processes based on performance metrics and feedback. Identify bottlenecks, inefficiencies, and areas for improvement. Regularly reviewing and updating processes ensures that the pharmacy remains efficient and responsive to changing needs.
- **Continuous Improvement Initiatives:** Implement continuous improvement initiatives, such as Lean or Six Sigma, to systematically identify and eliminate waste, streamline processes, and enhance overall efficiency. Encourage a culture of continuous improvement where staff are empowered to suggest and implement changes.

Enhancing Patient Experience

Optimizing workflow not only improves operational efficiency but also enhances the patient experience.

- **Patient-Centered Services:** Design workflow processes that prioritize patient convenience and satisfaction. For example, offer services such as medication synchronization, home delivery, and drive-thru pickups to meet patients' needs.
- **Clear Communication with Patients:** Provide clear and timely communication to patients regarding their prescriptions. Use automated systems to send text or email notifications when prescriptions are ready for pickup. Clear signage and information boards in the pharmacy can help guide patients and reduce confusion.
- **Personalized Care:** Ensure that patients receive personalized attention and care. Take the time to address their questions, provide counseling on medication use, and offer additional health services, such as immunizations or health screenings. A positive patient experience fosters loyalty and enhances the pharmacy's reputation.

Conclusion

Optimizing workflow in pharmacy settings involves a multifaceted approach that includes designing an effective layout, segmenting tasks, leveraging technology, ensuring efficient communication, managing workload, providing training, and continuously improving processes. By implementing these strategies, pharmacies can achieve greater efficiency, accuracy, and patient satisfaction.

As a pharmacy technician, your role in optimizing workflow is crucial. By adhering to best practices, staying informed about new technologies and methods, and actively contributing to continuous improvement efforts, you help create a more efficient and responsive pharmacy environment. This commitment to excellence ensures that patients receive the highest quality of care and that the pharmacy operates smoothly and effectively.

6. Pharmacy Financial Management

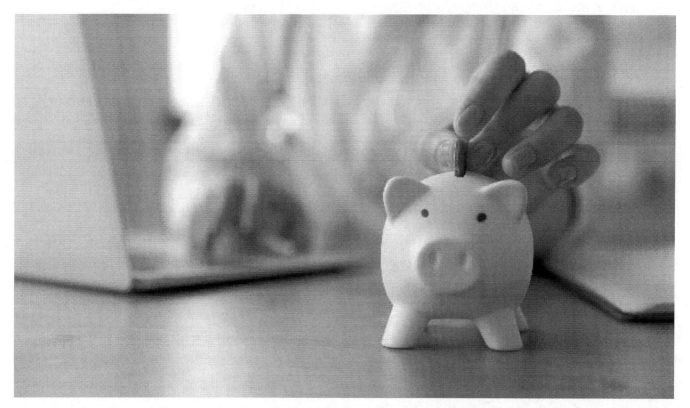

Managing the financial aspects of a pharmacy is much like tending to the intricate gears of a well-oiled machine. It requires a keen eye for detail, strategic thinking, and a thorough understanding of both the macro and microeconomic factors at play. In this chapter, we will delve into the essential components of pharmacy financial management, exploring how to navigate billing, insurance claims, reimbursement strategies, and audit processes.

Imagine you are at the helm of a busy pharmacy, balancing the books while ensuring that patients receive their medications promptly and efficiently. Financial management is not just about keeping the numbers in check; it's about creating a sustainable business model that supports excellent patient care. We'll uncover the strategies to maximize revenue, minimize costs, and maintain compliance with regulatory requirements.

Whether you are a seasoned pharmacy technician or new to the field, understanding these financial principles will empower you to contribute more effectively to your pharmacy's success. By mastering these concepts, you will be better equipped to support the financial health of the pharmacy, ensuring it can continue to provide vital services to the community. Let's embark on this journey to demystify the complexities of pharmacy financial management and discover how sound financial practices underpin a thriving pharmacy operation.

Basics of Billing in Pharmacy

Understanding the basics of billing in pharmacy is crucial for ensuring the financial health of the business and maintaining smooth operations. Effective billing practices not only ensure that the pharmacy is reimbursed for the services and medications provided but also help in building a reputation for reliability and efficiency. Let's delve into the key elements of pharmacy billing, exploring the process from the initial prescription to final payment.

The Billing Cycle

The billing cycle in a pharmacy begins when a prescription is received and ends when payment is collected. Each step in this cycle is vital for accurate and timely reimbursement.

Imagine a busy afternoon at the pharmacy. A patient comes in with a prescription from their doctor. This prescription initiates the billing process. The first step is data entry, where all relevant information from the prescription is entered into the pharmacy's information system. This includes the patient's details, the prescribed medication, dosage, and the prescribing physician's information. Accuracy at this stage is critical, as any errors can lead to delays or denials in payment.

Insurance Verification

Once the prescription information is entered, the next step is to verify the patient's insurance coverage. This process involves checking the patient's insurance details to confirm that the prescribed medication is covered under their plan. Insurance verification can sometimes be complex, with different insurers having varying requirements and formularies.

During verification, the pharmacy technician may need to contact the insurance provider to confirm details such as co-pays, deductibles, and any prior authorization requirements. This step ensures that the patient is aware of their financial responsibility and that the pharmacy can proceed with dispensing the medication without unexpected payment issues.

Claims Submission

After verifying the insurance coverage, the pharmacy submits a claim to the insurance provider. This claim includes all the necessary information about the prescription and the patient. The claim must be accurate and complete to avoid rejections or delays.

Claims are typically submitted electronically through the pharmacy's information system, which connects to the insurer's processing system. The electronic submission process is designed to be fast and efficient, reducing the time it takes for the claim to be reviewed and processed. However, it's essential to follow the specific formatting and coding requirements set by the insurer to ensure the claim is accepted.

Adjudication Process

Once the claim is submitted, it undergoes adjudication by the insurance provider. During adjudication, the insurer reviews the claim to determine its validity, the amount payable, and any patient responsibilities such as co-pays or deductibles.

This process involves checking the claim against the patient's insurance plan, the medication's coverage status, and any applicable formularies or restrictions. The insurer may approve the claim as submitted, approve it with modifications, or deny it. If the claim is denied, the pharmacy will need to investigate the reason for the denial and take appropriate action, such as correcting errors or providing additional documentation.

Reimbursement and Payment Collection

After the claim is adjudicated, the insurance provider reimburses the pharmacy for the approved amount. This reimbursement is typically deposited electronically into the pharmacy's bank account. The patient is responsible for paying any remaining balance, such as co-pays or deductibles.

Collecting payment from patients can sometimes be challenging, especially if they are unaware of their financial responsibilities. Effective communication and clear billing statements can help ensure that patients understand their obligations and make timely payments. Offering multiple payment options, such as credit cards, electronic payments, and installment plans, can also facilitate payment collection.

Handling Denials and Rejections

Despite best efforts, not all claims are accepted on the first submission. Denials and rejections are a common part of the billing process, and handling them efficiently is crucial for maintaining cash flow. When a claim is denied, the pharmacy must determine the reason for the denial and take corrective action. Common reasons for denials include incorrect patient information, coding errors, and lack of prior authorization. By promptly addressing these issues, the pharmacy can resubmit the claim and increase the likelihood of approval.

Rejections, on the other hand, typically occur at the initial submission stage and are often due to formatting or data entry errors. These can usually be corrected quickly and the claim resubmitted without significant delays.

Billing for Additional Services

Modern pharmacies offer a range of services beyond dispensing medications, such as immunizations, medication therapy management (MTM), and health screenings. Billing for these services requires understanding the specific codes and requirements associated with each service.

For example, billing for immunizations involves including the appropriate vaccine administration codes along with the medication code. MTM services may require documentation of the time spent and the specific interventions provided. Ensuring accurate and comprehensive documentation is essential for successful reimbursement for these additional services.

Maintaining Compliance

Compliance with federal, state, and insurer-specific regulations is a critical aspect of pharmacy billing. Non-compliance can result in denied claims, financial penalties, and damage to the pharmacy's reputation.

Key compliance areas include following the guidelines set by the Centers for Medicare & Medicaid Services (CMS), adhering to the Health Insurance Portability and Accountability Act (HIPAA) for patient privacy, and meeting state-specific regulations for pharmacy practice. Staying informed about changes in regulations and regularly auditing billing practices can help ensure ongoing compliance.

Utilizing Technology

Technology plays a significant role in streamlining the billing process and reducing errors. Pharmacy information systems (PIS) automate many aspects of billing, from claim submission to payment tracking.

Using a PIS with integrated billing capabilities can simplify the process of entering prescription details, verifying insurance coverage, and submitting claims. Additionally, these systems can generate reports that provide insights into billing performance, highlight trends, and identify areas for improvement.

Electronic health records (EHR) integration further enhances billing efficiency by ensuring that patient information is accurate and up-to-date. This reduces the likelihood of errors and improves the accuracy of claims submitted to insurers.

Staff Training and Development

Effective billing requires knowledgeable and skilled staff who understand the complexities of the process. Regular training and development programs ensure that pharmacy technicians and billing specialists stay current with best practices, regulatory changes, and new technologies.

Training should cover all aspects of the billing cycle, including data entry, insurance verification, claims submission, and handling denials. Providing opportunities for staff to attend workshops, webinars, and certification programs can enhance their skills and contribute to more efficient billing practices.

Mastering the basics of billing in pharmacy is essential for ensuring the financial health of the business and providing high-quality patient care. By understanding each step of the billing cycle, from prescription intake to payment collection, and implementing best practices for handling denials, maintaining compliance, and utilizing technology, pharmacies can optimize their billing processes.

Effective billing practices not only ensure timely reimbursement but also enhance the overall efficiency and reputation of the pharmacy. As a pharmacy technician, your role in the billing process is crucial, and by staying informed and engaged, you can contribute to the success and sustainability of the pharmacy. This commitment to excellence in billing reflects the broader goal of delivering reliable, high-quality pharmaceutical services to the community.

NAVIGATING COMPLEX INSURANCE CLAIMS

Navigating complex insurance claims is a critical skill for pharmacy technicians, requiring a blend of knowledge, patience, and meticulous attention to detail. Successfully managing these claims ensures that the pharmacy is reimbursed accurately and timely, and it also helps in maintaining positive relationships with patients and insurance providers. Let's explore the intricacies of handling complex insurance claims, from understanding insurance policies to resolving claim denials and appeals.

Understanding Insurance Policies

The foundation of navigating complex insurance claims begins with a thorough understanding of various insurance policies. Each insurance plan has its own set of rules, coverage limits, formularies, and authorization requirements.

Imagine a patient arrives with a prescription for a specialty medication. The first step is to verify the insurance coverage. This involves checking the patient's insurance card and accessing the pharmacy's information system to understand the specifics of their plan. Key details to look for include the formulary (the list of medications covered by the insurance plan), co-pays, deductibles, and any prior authorization requirements.

Formularies and Coverage

Formularies play a crucial role in determining which medications are covered by an insurance plan. These lists are typically divided into tiers, with each tier representing different levels of coverage and patient cost-sharing.

For example, a tier 1 medication might have a low co-pay, while a tier 3 medication could require a higher co-pay or even full payment if not covered. Understanding these tiers helps in guiding patients about their financial responsibilities and exploring alternatives if a prescribed medication is not covered.

In cases where a prescribed medication is not on the formulary, you might need to contact the prescribing physician to discuss alternative medications that are covered or initiate a prior authorization request to justify the necessity of the non-formulary medication.

Prior Authorization

Prior authorization (PA) is a process where the insurance provider requires additional information before approving coverage for certain medications. This step is often necessary for high-cost medications or treatments that are not on the formulary.

To obtain a prior authorization, you need to gather relevant clinical information and documentation from the prescribing physician. This may include medical history, diagnostic tests, and a rationale for why the specific medication is necessary. The PA request is then submitted to the insurance provider for review.

Navigating the PA process can be time-consuming, but it is essential for ensuring that patients receive the medications they need without incurring unexpected costs. Keeping detailed records and following up regularly with the insurance provider can help expedite the approval process.

Handling Claim Denials

Despite careful planning and verification, claim denials are a common occurrence in the pharmacy. Understanding how to handle these denials effectively is crucial for maintaining cash flow and patient satisfaction.

When a claim is denied, the first step is to understand the reason for the denial. Common reasons include incorrect patient information, missing documentation, non-covered medications, and lack of prior authorization. The denial notice from the insurance provider will usually specify the reason.

Once the reason for the denial is identified, you can take corrective action. This might involve updating patient information, providing additional documentation, or contacting the prescribing physician to discuss alternative medications. Resubmitting the corrected claim promptly increases the chances of approval.

Appealing Denied Claims

In cases where a claim is denied despite all required documentation and procedures being followed, an appeal may be necessary. The appeals process allows the pharmacy to present additional information and argue the case for why the medication should be covered.

The first step in the appeals process is to gather all relevant information, including the initial claim, denial notice, and supporting documentation. A well-organized appeal letter that clearly outlines the reasons for the appeal, supported by clinical evidence and physician statements, can strengthen the case.

It's important to adhere to the insurance provider's timelines and procedures for filing an appeal. Regular follow-up with the insurance provider ensures that the appeal is being reviewed and that any additional information requested is provided promptly.

Coordination of Benefits

Patients with multiple insurance plans require coordination of benefits (COB) to determine the primary and secondary payers. Proper coordination ensures that the pharmacy receives the maximum reimbursement while minimizing out-of-pocket costs for the patient.

When processing claims for patients with multiple insurance plans, verify each plan's details and determine which plan is primary. The primary insurance is billed first, and any remaining balance is submitted to the secondary insurance. Accurate data entry and clear communication with both insurance providers are essential for successful COB.

Navigating Specialty Medications

Specialty medications, which often include biologics and high-cost treatments, require a more complex claims process. These medications typically have stringent authorization requirements and may need to be sourced from specialty pharmacies.

Handling specialty medication claims involves close collaboration with the prescribing physician, the patient, and the insurance provider. Detailed documentation and regular follow-up are crucial to ensure that the necessary approvals are obtained and that the medication is delivered to the patient in a timely manner.

Patient Assistance Programs

For patients who struggle to afford their medications, patient assistance programs (PAPs) and manufacturer co-pay assistance can provide financial relief. These programs often require detailed applications and supporting documentation.

As a pharmacy technician, assisting patients with PAPs involves identifying eligible programs, helping patients complete applications, and coordinating with program administrators. This support can make a significant difference in ensuring that patients receive their medications without financial hardship.

Maintaining Compliance

Compliance with insurance regulations and policies is essential to avoid legal and financial repercussions. Regular training and staying informed about changes in insurance guidelines help ensure that billing practices remain compliant.

Maintain accurate and thorough records of all claims, denials, appeals, and communications with insurance providers. Regular audits and reviews of billing practices help identify areas for improvement and ensure that the pharmacy is adhering to best practices.

Building Relationships

Building strong relationships with insurance providers, physicians, and patients is key to navigating complex insurance claims successfully. Clear communication and collaboration foster trust and facilitate the resolution of issues.

Regularly updating physicians on the status of prior authorizations and appeals, keeping patients informed about their coverage and financial responsibilities, and maintaining open lines of communication with insurance providers help create a cooperative environment that supports efficient claims processing.

Navigating complex insurance claims is a multifaceted process that requires a deep understanding of insurance policies, meticulous attention to detail, and effective communication skills. By mastering the intricacies of formularies, prior authorizations, claim denials, and appeals, pharmacy technicians play a crucial role in ensuring that patients receive their medications without unnecessary delays or financial burdens.

Effective management of insurance claims not only enhances the financial health of the pharmacy but also builds trust and satisfaction among patients and healthcare providers. By staying informed, maintaining compliance, and fostering collaborative relationships, pharmacy technicians can navigate the complexities of insurance claims with confidence and expertise, ensuring a smooth and efficient operation that benefits all stakeholders.

STRATEGIES FOR EFFECTIVE REIMBURSEMENT

Effective reimbursement is crucial for the financial health and sustainability of a pharmacy. Ensuring timely and accurate reimbursement requires a blend of strategic planning, meticulous documentation, and proactive communication with insurance providers. In this subchapter, we will explore strategies that can enhance reimbursement processes, from understanding payer requirements to leveraging technology and optimizing billing practices.

Understanding Payer Requirements

The first step in achieving effective reimbursement is understanding the specific requirements of different payers, including private insurance companies, Medicare, and Medicaid. Each payer has its own set of rules, documentation requirements, and timelines.

Start by familiarizing yourself with the formularies, coverage policies, and reimbursement rates of the major insurers your pharmacy works with. This knowledge allows you to anticipate potential issues and prepare accordingly. For instance, some insurers might require prior authorization for certain medications or limit the quantity dispensed per month. Knowing these details upfront can prevent claim rejections and delays.

Comprehensive Documentation

Accurate and comprehensive documentation is the cornerstone of successful reimbursement. Detailed records ensure that all necessary information is available to support claims, reducing the likelihood of denials and facilitating smoother processing.

Every prescription should be accompanied by complete documentation, including the patient's medical history, diagnosis, and justification for the prescribed medication. This is particularly important for high-cost or specialty medications that often require additional scrutiny from insurers.

Documentation should also include any communication with the prescriber regarding the necessity of the medication, as well as any steps taken to comply with payer requirements, such as obtaining prior authorization. Maintaining thorough records not only supports reimbursement but also ensures compliance with regulatory requirements.

Efficient Claims Submission

Timely and accurate submission of claims is essential for effective reimbursement. Implementing efficient claims submission processes helps ensure that claims are processed without unnecessary delays.

Utilize electronic claim submission whenever possible, as this method is faster and more reliable than manual submission. Electronic claims are less prone to errors and can be tracked more easily through the payer's system. Ensure that all required fields are completed accurately and that the claim is formatted according to the payer's specifications.

Regularly review submission guidelines from each payer to stay current with any changes in their requirements. Submitting claims correctly the first time reduces the likelihood of rejections and the need for resubmission.

Managing Denials and Rejections

Despite best efforts, some claims may be denied or rejected. Effective management of these situations is crucial for maintaining cash flow and ensuring reimbursement.

When a claim is denied, promptly investigate the reason for the denial. Common reasons include missing information, incorrect coding, or failure to obtain prior authorization. Address these issues quickly and resubmit the claim with the necessary corrections.

For rejected claims, review the rejection notice to understand the specific error. Often, rejections are due to simple mistakes such as incorrect patient information or missing data. Correct these errors and resubmit the claim promptly.

Implementing a systematic approach to managing denials and rejections, including regular follow-up with payers, can significantly improve reimbursement rates. Tracking the status of all claims and maintaining clear records of communications with payers helps streamline this process.

Optimizing Coding Practices

Accurate coding is essential for ensuring that claims are processed correctly and reimbursed promptly. Coding errors are a common cause of claim denials and can significantly impact reimbursement.

Ensure that all pharmacy staff involved in the billing process are trained in the correct use of Current Procedural Terminology (CPT), Healthcare Common Procedure Coding System (HCPCS), and National Drug Codes (NDC). Regular training sessions and updates on coding changes can help maintain accuracy.

Implement checks and balances within the billing process to verify that the correct codes are used for each claim. This includes double-checking codes against the patient's diagnosis and the prescribed medication. Utilizing coding software or tools that integrate with your pharmacy information system can also enhance accuracy.

Leveraging Technology

Technology plays a vital role in optimizing reimbursement processes. Leveraging advanced billing and pharmacy management systems can streamline operations and improve accuracy.

Pharmacy information systems (PIS) with integrated billing modules can automate many aspects of the reimbursement process, from claim submission to payment tracking. These systems reduce manual errors and provide real-time insights into the status of claims.

Electronic health records (EHR) integration enhances the flow of information between healthcare providers and the pharmacy, ensuring that all necessary documentation is available for billing. This integration supports efficient claims submission and reduces the likelihood of missing information.

Analytics tools can also be invaluable for identifying trends and areas for improvement in the reimbursement process. By analyzing data on claim denials, rejections, and payment timelines, pharmacies can pinpoint issues and implement targeted strategies to enhance reimbursement.

Proactive Communication

Maintaining proactive communication with both payers and patients is essential for effective reimbursement. Clear communication helps prevent misunderstandings and ensures that all parties are aware of their responsibilities.

Establish regular contact with payer representatives to stay informed about changes in policies and procedures. This relationship can also be beneficial when resolving issues with specific claims. Being proactive in communication can expedite the resolution of problems and improve overall reimbursement rates.

For patients, clear communication about their insurance coverage, co-pays, and any out-of-pocket expenses is crucial. Providing patients with detailed explanations and answering their questions promptly can prevent confusion and ensure that they fulfill their financial responsibilities.

Training and Education

Continuous training and education for pharmacy staff are critical for maintaining effective reimbursement practices. Keeping staff informed about the latest billing regulations, payer requirements, and coding practices ensures that they are equipped to handle complex claims efficiently.

Regular training sessions on billing procedures, claim submission, and denial management help reinforce best practices and reduce the likelihood of errors. Encouraging staff to pursue certifications in billing and coding can also enhance their expertise and contribute to improved reimbursement rates.

Monitoring and Improving Performance

Continuous monitoring and improvement of reimbursement practices are essential for maintaining financial health. Implementing performance metrics and regularly reviewing these metrics help identify areas for improvement and track progress over time.

Key performance indicators (KPIs) for reimbursement might include claim acceptance rates, denial rates, time to payment, and overall reimbursement amounts. Analyzing these metrics can highlight inefficiencies and guide targeted improvements.

Conduct regular audits of billing practices to ensure compliance with payer requirements and regulatory standards. These audits can also identify training needs and areas where processes can be optimized.

Conclusion

Effective reimbursement is a complex but vital aspect of pharmacy financial management. By understanding payer requirements, maintaining comprehensive documentation, optimizing coding practices, leveraging technology, and fostering proactive communication, pharmacies can enhance their reimbursement processes.

Training and continuous improvement are essential for ensuring that staff are equipped to handle the complexities of billing and reimbursement. By implementing these strategies, pharmacies can improve their financial stability and continue to provide high-quality care to their patients. As a pharmacy technician, mastering these practices will enable you to contribute significantly to the financial success and operational efficiency of your pharmacy, ensuring that it remains a trusted and reliable resource for the community.

HANDLING AUDITS AND COMPLIANCE IN PHARMACY PRACTICE

Handling audits and maintaining compliance are critical aspects of pharmacy practice. They ensure that the pharmacy operates within legal and regulatory frameworks, maintains high standards of patient care, and safeguards its financial health. This subchapter explores the intricacies of managing audits and ensuring compliance, from understanding regulatory requirements to preparing for audits and implementing effective compliance strategies.

Understanding Regulatory Requirements

The foundation of effective audit and compliance management lies in a thorough understanding of the regulatory environment. Pharmacies are subject to a complex web of federal, state, and local regulations designed to ensure the safe and effective dispensing of medications.

Key federal regulations include those enforced by the Drug Enforcement Administration (DEA), the Food and Drug Administration (FDA), and the Centers for Medicare & Medicaid Services (CMS).

These agencies set standards for the handling of controlled substances, the quality and safety of medications, and the billing practices for Medicare and Medicaid.

State pharmacy boards also impose regulations that govern pharmacy operations, including licensing requirements, staffing ratios, and record-keeping practices. Staying informed about these regulations and any changes is essential for maintaining compliance.

Preparing for Audits

Audits are a routine part of pharmacy practice, conducted by regulatory agencies, insurance companies, and internal teams to ensure compliance with laws and policies. Preparation is key to a successful audit, and it begins with maintaining accurate and comprehensive records.

1. **Documentation:** Ensure that all records, including prescription logs, inventory records, billing documents, and patient files, are complete, accurate, and up-to-date. Proper documentation provides a clear trail of all pharmacy activities and transactions.

2. **Training:** Regularly train staff on audit procedures and compliance requirements. Ensure that everyone understands their role in maintaining compliance and knows how to respond to audit requests.

3. **Mock Audits:** Conduct internal mock audits to identify potential issues and areas for improvement. These practice audits help staff become familiar with the audit process and highlight any gaps in compliance that need to be addressed.

4. **Organized Record-Keeping:** Develop an organized system for storing and retrieving records. Easy access to documentation ensures that auditors can review the necessary information quickly and efficiently.

Conducting Internal Audits

Internal audits are proactive measures that help identify and rectify compliance issues before they become significant problems. These audits should be conducted regularly and cover all aspects of pharmacy operations.

1. **Compliance Checklist:** Develop a comprehensive compliance checklist that includes all regulatory requirements and internal policies. Use this checklist as a guide during internal audits to ensure that all areas are reviewed.

2. **Inventory Management:** Regularly audit inventory records to ensure accurate tracking of medications, especially controlled substances. Discrepancies between physical inventory and records can indicate issues such as theft, loss, or improper record-keeping.

3. **Billing and Claims:** Review billing practices and submitted claims to ensure accuracy and compliance with payer requirements. Look for patterns of denied claims or billing errors that need to be addressed.

4. **Record Accuracy:** Verify that all patient records, prescription logs, and documentation are accurate and complete. Incomplete or inaccurate records can lead to compliance violations and audit failures.

Responding to External Audits

When notified of an external audit, it's important to respond promptly and cooperate fully with auditors. Preparation and organization are key to a smooth audit process.

1. **Audit Notification:** Upon receiving notification of an audit, review the scope and requirements of the audit. Assign a point person to coordinate the audit process and serve as the main contact for auditors.

2. **Gathering Documents:** Collect all requested documents and ensure they are complete and well-organized. Provide auditors with easy access to records and be prepared to answer any questions they may have.

3. **Transparency:** Maintain transparency and honesty throughout the audit process. If any issues or discrepancies are identified, address them openly and provide explanations or corrective actions as needed.

4. **Follow-Up:** After the audit, review the auditor's findings and take corrective actions as necessary. Address any identified compliance issues promptly and implement measures to prevent future occurrences.

Maintaining Ongoing Compliance

Compliance is not a one-time effort but an ongoing process that requires continuous attention and improvement. Implementing effective compliance strategies helps ensure that the pharmacy remains compliant with all regulatory requirements.

1. **Regular Training:** Continuously educate staff on compliance requirements and best practices. Regular training sessions help keep everyone informed about changes in regulations and reinforce the importance of compliance.

2. **Compliance Officer:** Designate a compliance officer or team responsible for overseeing compliance efforts. This individual or team should stay up-to-date with regulatory changes, conduct regular audits, and provide guidance on compliance matters.

3. **Policy Development:** Develop and regularly update comprehensive policies and procedures that address all aspects of pharmacy operations. Ensure that these policies are communicated to all staff and are easily accessible.

4. **Risk Management:** Implement a risk management program to identify and mitigate potential compliance risks. Regularly assess the pharmacy's operations and address any vulnerabilities that could lead to compliance violations.

Leveraging Technology

Technology can play a significant role in maintaining compliance and managing audits. Utilizing advanced pharmacy management systems and compliance software enhances accuracy and efficiency.

1. **Electronic Health Records (EHR):** Integrate EHR systems to ensure accurate and complete patient records. EHRs provide a comprehensive view of patient history, medications, and interactions, supporting compliance with documentation requirements.

2. **Automated Inventory Systems:** Use automated inventory management systems to track medications and control inventory levels. These systems provide real-time data and alerts for discrepancies, reducing the risk of errors and non-compliance.

3. **Billing Software:** Implement billing software that automates claim submission and tracks the status of claims. This software helps ensure that billing practices comply with payer requirements and reduces the likelihood of errors.

4. **Compliance Tracking Tools:** Utilize compliance tracking tools to monitor adherence to regulatory requirements. These tools can generate reports, track training and certification, and provide alerts for upcoming compliance deadlines.

Staying Informed

Staying informed about regulatory changes and industry developments is crucial for maintaining compliance. Regularly reviewing industry publications, attending conferences, and participating in professional organizations help keep you up-to-date with the latest information.

1. **Industry Publications:** Subscribe to industry publications and newsletters that provide updates on regulatory changes, best practices, and compliance tips. Staying informed helps you anticipate and prepare for changes that may impact your pharmacy.

2. **Professional Organizations:** Join professional organizations such as the American Pharmacists Association (APhA) or the National Community Pharmacists Association (NCPA). These organizations offer resources, training, and networking opportunities that support compliance efforts.

3. **Continuing Education:** Participate in continuing education programs to enhance your knowledge and skills. Many regulatory bodies require ongoing education as part of their compliance standards, ensuring that you remain informed and competent in your role.

Conclusion

Handling audits and maintaining compliance are essential responsibilities for any pharmacy. By understanding regulatory requirements, preparing thoroughly for audits, conducting regular internal reviews, and leveraging technology, pharmacies can ensure compliance and avoid the pitfalls of regulatory violations.

Effective compliance management not only protects the pharmacy from legal and financial risks but also enhances the quality of care provided to patients. As a pharmacy technician, your role in maintaining compliance is critical. By staying informed, organized, and proactive, you can contribute significantly to the pharmacy's success and its commitment to providing safe and effective healthcare services.

7. INTERPERSONAL ASPECTS OF PHARMACY WORK

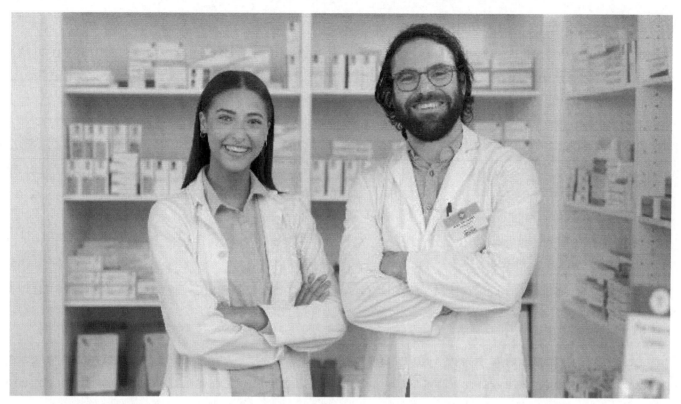

The role of a pharmacy technician extends far beyond managing medications and handling prescriptions. At the heart of this profession lies a vital human element: the interactions with patients, healthcare providers, and colleagues. The interpersonal aspects of pharmacy work are crucial in building trust, ensuring patient safety, and fostering a collaborative environment.

Imagine the daily rhythm of a pharmacy, where each interaction offers an opportunity to make a meaningful impact. From providing compassionate care to patients who may be anxious or unwell, to collaborating with a team of healthcare professionals, these moments define the essence of pharmacy practice. Effective communication, empathy, and professional relationships are the keystones of success in this field.

In this chapter, we will explore the various facets of interpersonal skills in pharmacy work. We'll delve into techniques for enhancing patient communication, strategies for managing sensitive patient data, and ways to improve patient care and safety. By mastering these skills, you'll not only enhance your professional capabilities but also contribute to a positive and supportive healthcare environment. Let's embark on this journey to understand how the human connection in pharmacy practice makes all the difference.

ENHANCING COMMUNICATION WITH PATIENTS

Enhancing communication with patients is one of the most impactful aspects of pharmacy work. Effective communication fosters trust, ensures that patients understand their medications, and improves adherence to treatment plans. This interaction is not just about exchanging information;

it's about connecting with patients, understanding their needs, and providing empathetic, personalized care.

Building Trust and Rapport

The foundation of effective communication with patients is trust. When patients trust their pharmacy team, they are more likely to share important information and follow their medication regimens. Building this trust begins with the first interaction and continues through every subsequent visit.

Imagine a patient walking into the pharmacy for the first time. Your warm greeting and attentive demeanor immediately set the tone for a positive interaction. Use the patient's name, maintain eye contact, and offer a friendly smile. These small gestures can make patients feel valued and respected.

Listening actively is another key component. When a patient speaks, give them your full attention. Nod to show understanding, and avoid interrupting. Reflect back what they have said to confirm your understanding and to show that you are listening. For example, "It sounds like you've been having trouble remembering to take your medication. Is that correct?"

Clarity and Simplicity in Communication

Patients come from diverse backgrounds and may have varying levels of health literacy. Therefore, it's crucial to communicate in a way that is clear and easy to understand. Avoid medical jargon and use simple language. When explaining how to take a medication, be specific and straightforward. Instead of saying, "Take this antihypertensive once daily," say, "Take this blood pressure pill once every morning."

Using visual aids can also enhance understanding. Show patients how to use inhalers, insulin pens, or other devices, and provide written instructions with diagrams. Repetition is another effective tool. Repeat key points and encourage patients to repeat instructions back to you to ensure they have understood correctly.

Empathy and Emotional Support

Empathy plays a crucial role in patient communication. Recognizing and addressing the emotional needs of patients can significantly enhance their overall experience. Many patients may feel anxious, frustrated, or overwhelmed by their health issues. Expressing empathy involves acknowledging these feelings and offering support.

For example, if a patient expresses concern about a new diagnosis, you might say, "I understand that this diagnosis can be overwhelming. Let's talk about your treatment plan and how we can manage it together." This approach not only provides emotional support but also encourages patients to take an active role in their healthcare.

Patient Education

Educating patients about their medications is a core responsibility of pharmacy technicians. Effective education involves more than just explaining how to take a medication; it also includes discussing why the medication is important, what to expect, and how to manage potential side effects.

When educating patients, tailor your approach to their specific needs and preferences. Some patients may prefer detailed explanations, while others might benefit from concise, focused information. Ask open-ended questions to gauge their understanding and address any concerns they might have. For instance, "What do you know about this medication?" or "Do you have any questions about how to take this medicine?"

Provide information about potential side effects and what to do if they occur. For example, "This medication might cause dizziness, especially when you first start taking it. If you feel dizzy, try sitting down until it passes, and let us know if it becomes a problem."

Encouraging Adherence

One of the significant challenges in pharmacy practice is ensuring that patients adhere to their prescribed treatment plans. Effective communication strategies can significantly improve adherence.

First, help patients understand the importance of taking their medications as prescribed. Explain how the medication works, the benefits of consistent use, and the risks of non-adherence. For example, "Taking this medication every day helps keep your blood pressure under control, reducing your risk of heart attacks and strokes."

Offer practical tips to help patients remember their medications. Suggest using pill organizers, setting alarms, or associating medication times with daily routines, such as brushing teeth. Regular follow-ups, either in person or through phone calls, can also reinforce adherence. Check in to see how they are managing and address any barriers they might be facing.

Cultural Sensitivity

Patients come from diverse cultural backgrounds, and understanding these cultural differences is essential for effective communication. Cultural sensitivity involves respecting and acknowledging these differences in beliefs, practices, and communication styles.

Take the time to learn about the cultural backgrounds of your patients and how these might influence their health behaviors and attitudes toward medication. For instance, some cultures may have specific beliefs about certain types of medications or treatments. Showing respect for these beliefs, while providing accurate information, can help build trust and encourage open communication.

Use language services, such as interpreters or translation tools, when necessary to ensure clear communication with patients who speak different languages. Providing written materials in multiple languages can also be helpful.

Using Technology to Enhance Communication

Technology offers numerous tools to enhance communication with patients. From automated reminders to telepharmacy services, these tools can improve accessibility and convenience for patients.

Automated text or phone reminders can help patients remember to take their medications or refill prescriptions. These reminders can be personalized to include specific instructions or motivational messages.

Telepharmacy services allow patients to consult with pharmacists remotely, which is especially beneficial for those with mobility issues or those living in remote areas. These virtual consultations can cover medication management, patient education, and adherence support.

Feedback and Continuous Improvement

Finally, seeking feedback from patients about their communication experiences can provide valuable insights and opportunities for improvement. Encourage patients to share their thoughts and experiences, either through surveys, suggestion boxes, or direct conversations.

Act on the feedback received to make necessary improvements. For example, if patients express difficulty understanding medication instructions, consider revising the educational materials or offering additional training for staff.

Conclusion

Enhancing communication with patients is a dynamic and ongoing process that requires empathy, clarity, and cultural sensitivity. By building trust, providing clear and concise information, offering emotional support, and using technology effectively, pharmacy technicians can significantly improve patient experiences and outcomes.

Effective communication not only ensures that patients understand their medications and adhere to their treatment plans but also fosters a positive and supportive healthcare environment. As a pharmacy technician, mastering these communication skills will enable you to make a meaningful difference in the lives of your patients, enhancing their health and well-being through compassionate and effective care.

TECHNIQUES FOR MANAGING SENSITIVE PATIENT DATA

Managing sensitive patient data is a crucial aspect of pharmacy practice, requiring meticulous attention to confidentiality, security, and regulatory compliance. The trust patients place in their pharmacy extends beyond medication management to include the safekeeping of their personal health information. Here, we explore effective techniques for managing sensitive patient data, ensuring privacy, and maintaining compliance with relevant laws and regulations.

Understanding Patient Confidentiality

Patient confidentiality is the cornerstone of trust in healthcare. It involves protecting patients' personal and medical information from unauthorized access and disclosure. Confidentiality is not just a legal obligation but a professional and ethical duty. When patients know their information is secure, they are more likely to share critical health details, enabling better care.

To ensure confidentiality, it's important to recognize the types of information that must be protected. This includes patient names, addresses, birth dates, social security numbers, medical histories, diagnoses, treatment plans, and medication details. Any information that can identify a patient and link them to their health data is considered sensitive.

HIPAA and Regulatory Compliance

In the United States, the Health Insurance Portability and Accountability Act (HIPAA) sets the standard for protecting sensitive patient information. HIPAA compliance involves adhering to rules regarding the use, disclosure, and safeguarding of protected health information (PHI). Understanding and implementing these regulations is crucial for all pharmacy staff.

HIPAA outlines several key requirements:

- **Privacy Rule:** This rule establishes national standards for the protection of PHI. It requires pharmacies to implement safeguards to protect the privacy of health information and to set limits on the use and disclosure of such information without patient authorization.
- **Security Rule:** This rule specifies administrative, physical, and technical safeguards to ensure the confidentiality, integrity, and availability of electronic PHI (ePHI). It mandates measures like access controls, encryption, and regular security assessments.
- **Breach Notification Rule:** This rule requires pharmacies to notify patients, the Department of Health and Human Services (HHS), and, in some cases, the media, of any breaches of unsecured PHI.

Implementing Administrative Safeguards

Administrative safeguards are policies and procedures designed to manage the selection, development, implementation, and maintenance of security measures to protect PHI. These safeguards also address workforce training and incident response.

1. **Policies and Procedures:** Develop comprehensive policies and procedures that outline how patient information is to be protected. These should cover aspects like data access, usage, storage, and disposal. Regularly review and update these policies to reflect changes in regulations and technology.
2. **Training and Education:** Regularly train all pharmacy staff on HIPAA requirements and the importance of protecting patient information. Training should cover recognizing potential breaches, proper data handling practices, and the consequences of non-compliance. Ongoing education ensures that staff stay informed about best practices and regulatory updates.
3. **Incident Response Plan:** Establish an incident response plan to address potential data breaches. This plan should include steps for identifying and containing breaches, notifying affected parties, and mitigating damage. Regularly test and update the plan to ensure its effectiveness.

Physical Safeguards

Physical safeguards involve measures to protect the physical security of patient information. These measures help prevent unauthorized access to facilities, equipment, and records.

1. **Secure Storage:** Ensure that all paper records and electronic devices containing PHI are stored securely. Use locked cabinets for physical records and restrict access to authorized personnel only. For electronic devices, use secure rooms or cabinets when not in use.
2. **Access Controls:** Implement access controls to restrict entry to areas where patient information is stored or processed. This includes using keycards, access codes, or biometric systems to limit access to authorized staff. Monitor access logs regularly to detect any unauthorized attempts.
3. **Workstation Security:** Position computer workstations in a way that prevents unauthorized viewing of patient information. Use privacy screens and ensure that

workstations automatically lock after a period of inactivity. Train staff to log out of systems when not in use.

Technical Safeguards

Technical safeguards are the technological measures used to protect ePHI. These safeguards ensure that patient information remains secure during transmission and storage.

1. **Encryption:** Encrypt ePHI both at rest and in transit. Encryption converts data into a coded format that can only be accessed by authorized users with the correct decryption key. This prevents unauthorized access to data, even if it is intercepted or stolen.

2. **Access Controls:** Implement role-based access controls to ensure that staff members can only access the information necessary for their job functions. Use strong, unique passwords and multi-factor authentication to enhance security.

3. **Audit Controls:** Use audit controls to monitor and log all access to and activities involving ePHI. Regularly review these logs to detect any suspicious activity or potential breaches. Audit logs provide a record of who accessed information and what actions they performed.

Secure Communication

Secure communication is vital when transmitting patient information between healthcare providers, insurance companies, and patients. Ensuring that these communications are protected prevents unauthorized access to sensitive information.

1. **Secure Messaging:** Use secure messaging systems for internal and external communications involving patient information. These systems encrypt messages and attachments, ensuring that only intended recipients can read them.

2. **Email Encryption:** When sending patient information via email, use encryption to protect the contents. Many email providers offer encryption services that can be easily integrated into daily workflows.

3. **Patient Portals:** Encourage patients to use secure patient portals for accessing their health information, communicating with the pharmacy, and managing prescriptions. These portals provide a secure platform for sharing sensitive information.

Data Minimization and Anonymization

Data minimization involves collecting and retaining only the information necessary for patient care and pharmacy operations. Anonymization removes personally identifiable information from data sets, reducing the risk if the data is accessed inappropriately.

1. **Limit Data Collection:** Only collect the information needed to fulfill a specific purpose. Avoid collecting excessive or irrelevant details that do not contribute to patient care.

2. **Anonymize Data:** When possible, use anonymized data for research, reporting, or other secondary purposes. Removing identifiable information protects patient privacy while allowing useful analysis.

Regular Audits and Assessments

Conducting regular audits and assessments helps ensure ongoing compliance with privacy and security standards. These evaluations identify vulnerabilities and areas for improvement.

1. **Internal Audits:** Perform regular internal audits to review compliance with HIPAA and other regulations. These audits should assess administrative, physical, and technical safeguards.

2. **Risk Assessments:** Conduct comprehensive risk assessments to identify potential threats to patient data. Evaluate the likelihood and impact of these threats and implement measures to mitigate them.

3. **Compliance Reviews:** Periodically review compliance with internal policies and procedures. Ensure that staff are following established guidelines and address any deviations promptly.

Patient Engagement and Transparency

Engaging patients in their own privacy protection and being transparent about how their information is used can build trust and enhance compliance efforts.

1. **Patient Education:** Educate patients about their rights under HIPAA and how their information is protected. Provide clear, accessible information about how data is collected, used, and shared.

2. **Privacy Notices:** Provide patients with a Notice of Privacy Practices that outlines how their information is handled and their rights regarding their data. Ensure that this notice is readily available and easy to understand.

3. **Feedback Mechanisms:** Establish mechanisms for patients to provide feedback or report concerns about their privacy. Address any issues raised promptly and transparently.

Managing sensitive patient data is a critical responsibility that requires a combination of administrative, physical, and technical safeguards. By understanding and implementing HIPAA regulations, maintaining comprehensive documentation, using secure communication methods, and engaging patients, pharmacy staff can protect patient information and build trust. Regular audits and continuous training ensure that these practices remain effective and up-to-date. As a pharmacy technician, your role in safeguarding patient data is crucial, contributing to the overall integrity and reliability of the pharmacy. Through diligent and informed practices, you help ensure that patient confidentiality is preserved and that the pharmacy operates in full compliance with all regulatory requirements.

IMPROVING PATIENT CARE AND SAFETY

Improving patient care and safety is at the heart of pharmacy practice. It's about ensuring that every patient receives the best possible care, which involves more than just dispensing medications accurately. It requires a proactive approach to patient interactions, education, and support, alongside rigorous safety protocols and continuous improvement efforts. Let's delve into the strategies and practices that can enhance patient care and safety in the pharmacy setting.

Building Strong Patient Relationships

The foundation of excellent patient care is building strong, trusting relationships with patients. This begins with effective communication and extends to every interaction.

When patients feel valued and understood, they are more likely to adhere to their medication regimens and follow health advice. Start by greeting each patient warmly, using their name, and showing genuine interest in their well-being. Listen actively to their concerns and questions, and provide clear, empathetic responses. Creating a welcoming environment encourages patients to engage more openly, sharing vital information that can aid in their care.

Patient Education and Empowerment

Educating patients about their medications and health conditions is a crucial aspect of patient care. An informed patient is better equipped to manage their health, leading to improved outcomes.

When dispensing medications, take the time to explain how the medication works, its benefits, potential side effects, and the importance of adherence. Use clear, simple language and avoid medical jargon. Providing written materials or visual aids can help reinforce verbal instructions. Encourage patients to ask questions and clarify any doubts they may have. For instance, you might say, "This medication helps control your blood pressure. It's important to take it every day at the same time to keep your levels stable. Do you have any questions about how to take it?"

Medication Therapy Management (MTM)

Medication Therapy Management (MTM) services are designed to optimize therapeutic outcomes for patients. These services include comprehensive medication reviews, identifying and resolving medication-related problems, and developing personalized care plans.

During an MTM session, review the patient's complete medication list, including prescription drugs, over-the-counter medications, and supplements. Look for potential drug interactions, duplications, or contraindications. Discuss any issues or side effects the patient is experiencing and collaborate with the prescribing physician to make necessary adjustments. MTM services not only improve medication safety but also enhance patient adherence and satisfaction.

Implementing Safety Protocols

Ensuring patient safety involves implementing rigorous protocols to prevent errors and adverse events. These protocols should cover all aspects of pharmacy operations, from prescription verification to medication dispensing.

1. **Prescription Verification:** Double-check each prescription for accuracy before dispensing. Verify the patient's name, medication, dosage, and instructions. If there are any discrepancies or uncertainties, contact the prescriber for clarification. Using technology, such as barcode scanning, can enhance the accuracy of this process.

2. **Patient Identification:** Always confirm the patient's identity before dispensing medications. Use at least two identifiers, such as name and date of birth, to ensure the right patient receives the right medication.

3. **Safe Dispensing Practices:** Follow best practices for medication dispensing, including using calibrated equipment for measuring doses and double-checking labels before finalizing

the prescription. Implementing a double-check system where another pharmacy technician or pharmacist reviews the prescription can further reduce errors.

Adherence Support

Medication adherence is a significant challenge in patient care. Providing support and resources to help patients stick to their treatment plans is essential.

1. **Reminder Systems:** Offer tools such as pill organizers, medication calendars, or mobile app reminders to help patients remember to take their medications. Setting up automatic refill reminders can also ensure that patients don't run out of their medications.

2. **Follow-Up:** Schedule follow-up calls or visits to check on the patient's progress and address any issues they may be facing. Regular follow-ups provide an opportunity to reinforce the importance of adherence and make any necessary adjustments to the treatment plan.

3. **Addressing Barriers:** Identify and address common barriers to adherence, such as side effects, cost, or forgetfulness. Work with patients to find solutions, such as switching to medications with fewer side effects, exploring generic alternatives, or setting up a convenient dosing schedule.

Collaborative Care

Collaboration with other healthcare providers is vital for comprehensive patient care. Effective communication and teamwork ensure that all aspects of the patient's health are addressed.

1. **Communication with Prescribers:** Maintain open lines of communication with physicians and other prescribers. Share relevant information about the patient's medication history, adherence, and any issues that arise. This collaboration helps in making informed decisions about the patient's treatment plan.

2. **Interdisciplinary Teams:** Participate in interdisciplinary care teams that include doctors, nurses, dietitians, and other healthcare professionals. These teams work together to develop and implement holistic care plans that address the patient's physical, emotional, and social needs.

3. **Referrals and Resources:** When necessary, refer patients to other healthcare providers or community resources for additional support. This might include referrals to specialists, support groups, or social services.

Continuous Improvement

Improving patient care and safety is an ongoing process that requires regular evaluation and adaptation. Implementing a culture of continuous improvement ensures that the pharmacy stays current with best practices and evolving patient needs.

1. **Quality Improvement Programs:** Establish quality improvement programs that regularly assess and enhance pharmacy practices. Use data and patient feedback to identify areas for improvement and implement changes. For example, if a pattern of medication errors is identified, analyze the root causes and develop strategies to prevent future occurrences.

2. **Staff Training:** Provide ongoing training and education for all pharmacy staff. This includes training on new medications, emerging health trends, and updated safety protocols.

Encouraging professional development helps staff stay informed and competent in their roles.

3. **Patient Feedback:** Actively seek and act on patient feedback. Use surveys, suggestion boxes, or direct conversations to gather input on their experiences. Addressing patient feedback helps improve service quality and patient satisfaction.

Technology and Innovation

Leveraging technology can significantly enhance patient care and safety. Innovations in pharmacy practice provide new tools and methods to improve efficiency and accuracy.

1. **Electronic Health Records (EHR):** Utilize EHR systems to maintain comprehensive patient records. EHRs facilitate better coordination of care and provide pharmacists with access to critical patient information, such as lab results and previous medication history.

2. **Telepharmacy:** Implement telepharmacy services to provide remote consultations and support. This is particularly useful for patients in rural or underserved areas who may have limited access to in-person pharmacy services.

3. **Automated Dispensing Systems:** Use automated dispensing systems to improve the accuracy and efficiency of medication dispensing. These systems reduce the risk of human error and streamline the workflow.

Improving patient care and safety in pharmacy practice is a multifaceted endeavor that requires a combination of strong interpersonal skills, rigorous safety protocols, and a commitment to continuous improvement. By building trust with patients, providing thorough education, supporting adherence, and collaborating with other healthcare providers, pharmacy technicians play a crucial role in enhancing patient outcomes.

Embracing technology and innovation further enhances the ability to provide safe and effective care. As a pharmacy technician, your dedication to these practices ensures that patients receive the highest standard of care, fostering a positive and supportive healthcare environment. Through these efforts, you contribute significantly to the well-being of your patients and the overall success of the pharmacy.

8. REFRESHER ON PHARMACY MATH BASICS

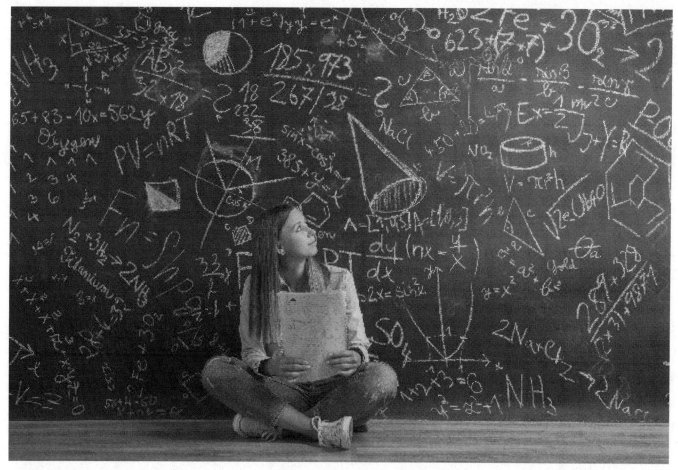

Mastering pharmacy math is fundamental for any pharmacy technician. From calculating correct dosages to preparing precise compounding formulas, a solid grasp of math ensures accuracy and safety in patient care. However, the intricacies of pharmacy calculations can sometimes be daunting, and even the most experienced professionals can benefit from a refresher.

In this chapter, we'll revisit the essential principles of pharmacy math. We'll start with the basics, such as understanding units of measurement and conversions, before delving into more complex calculations required in everyday practice. Imagine preparing a complex medication regimen for a pediatric patient or calculating the precise amount of a compound for an intravenous infusion. These tasks require not only theoretical knowledge but also practical problem-solving skills and attention to detail.

By reinforcing these foundational math skills, you'll enhance your confidence and competence in handling various pharmaceutical calculations. This chapter aims to make math approachable and applicable, using real-world examples to illustrate each concept. Whether you're refreshing your knowledge or filling in gaps, this comprehensive review will equip you with the tools you need to excel in your role and ensure the highest standards of patient care.

DETAILED CALCULATIONS FOR DRUG DOSAGES

Calculating drug dosages accurately is a critical skill for pharmacy technicians. Whether adjusting doses for pediatric patients, compounding medications, or preparing intravenous infusions, precise calculations are essential for patient safety and effective treatment. In this subchapter, we will explore the methods and principles behind detailed drug dosage calculations, using real-world examples to illustrate these concepts.

Basic Principles of Dosage Calculations

The foundation of dosage calculations lies in understanding the relationship between the dose, the concentration of the drug, and the volume required. The basic formula often used is:

$$\text{Dose} = \text{Concentration} \times \text{Volume}$$

This equation helps determine how much of a drug is needed based on its strength and the desired dose. Let's break down each component to understand how they interact.

Unit Conversions

One of the most common tasks in pharmacy math is converting units. This might involve converting milligrams to grams, milliliters to liters, or adjusting for different measurement systems. It's crucial to ensure that all units are consistent before performing any calculations.

For example, if a prescription calls for 500 mg of a medication, and the available drug concentration is 250 mg per 5 mL, you need to convert and calculate the required volume:

$$\text{Volume} = \frac{\text{Dose}}{\text{Concentration}} = \frac{500 \text{ mg}}{250 \text{ mg/5 mL}} = \frac{500}{250} \times 5 \text{ mL} = 10 \text{ mL}$$

Weight-Based Dosage Calculations

Weight-based dosing is common, especially in pediatrics and oncology, where dosages must be carefully tailored to the patient's weight. The formula for weight-based dosages is:

$$\text{Dose} = \text{Patient's Weight (kg)} \times \text{Dose per kg}$$

For instance, if a medication requires a dose of 2 mg/kg for a patient weighing 30 kg, the calculation would be:

$$\text{Dose} = 30 \text{ kg} \times 2 \text{ mg/kg} = 60 \text{ mg}$$

If the medication is available in a concentration of 10 mg/mL, the volume needed would be:

$$\text{Volume} = \frac{60 \text{ mg}}{10 \text{ mg/mL}} = 6 \text{ mL}$$

Body Surface Area (BSA) Calculations

In oncology and some other specialties, dosages are often calculated based on body surface area (BSA). The Mosteller formula is a commonly used method to estimate BSA:

$$\text{BSA(m}^2) = \sqrt{\frac{\text{Height (cm)} \times \text{Weight (kg)}}{3600}}$$

For example, for a patient who is 150 cm tall and weighs 50 kg:

$$\text{BSA} = \sqrt{\frac{150 \times 50}{3600}} = \sqrt{\frac{7500}{3600}} \approx 1.29 \text{ m}^2$$

If the prescribed medication dose is 150 mg/m22, the total dose would be:

$$\text{Total Dose} = 1.29 \text{ m}^2 \times 150 \text{ mg/m}^2 = 193.5 \text{ mg}$$

Intravenous (IV) Infusion Calculations

IV infusions require precise calculations to ensure the correct rate of drug administration. The key formula for calculating the infusion rate is:

$$\text{Infusion Rate} = \frac{\text{Volume (mL)}}{\text{Time (hours)}}$$

For example, if an IV medication needs to be administered at a dose of 200 mg over 4 hours, and the drug concentration is 50 mg/mL, first calculate the volume:

$$\text{Volume} = \frac{200 \text{ mg}}{50 \text{ mg/mL}} = 4 \text{ mL}$$

Then, calculate the infusion rate:

$$\text{Infusion Rate} = \frac{4 \text{ mL}}{4 \text{ hours}} = 1 \text{ mL/hour}$$

Adjusting for Patient-Specific Factors

Certain patient-specific factors, such as renal or hepatic impairment, can affect drug dosing. Adjusting doses for these conditions is critical to avoid toxicity or subtherapeutic effects.

For example, a patient with reduced renal function may require a lower dose of a renally-excreted drug. If the standard dose is 100 mg but needs to be reduced by 50% due to renal impairment, the adjusted dose would be:

$$\text{Adjusted Dose} = 100 \text{ mg} \times 0.5 = 50 \text{ mg}$$

Practical Example: Pediatric Dosing

Pediatric dosing often requires extra caution and precision. Consider a scenario where a child weighing 20 kg needs a medication dosed at 10 mg/kg/day, divided into two doses.

First, calculate the total daily dose:

$$\text{Total Daily Dose} = 20 \text{ kg} \times 10 \text{ mg/kg/day} = 200 \text{ mg/day}$$

Next, determine the dose per administration (since it's divided into two doses):

$$\text{Dose per Administration} = \frac{200 \text{ mg/day}}{2} = 100 \text{ mg}$$

If the medication is available in a syrup form with a concentration of 25 mg/5 mL, calculate the volume per dose:

$$\text{Volume per Dose} = \frac{100 \text{ mg}}{25 \text{ mg/5 mL}} = \frac{100}{25} \times 5 \text{ mL} = 20 \text{ mL}$$

Practical Example: Compounding a Cream

Compounding requires precise measurements to ensure the correct concentration of active ingredients. Suppose you need to prepare 50 grams of a 2% hydrocortisone cream.

First, calculate the amount of hydrocortisone needed:

$$\text{Hydrocortisone Amount} = 50 \text{ g} \times 0.02 = 1 \text{ g}$$

You will then incorporate 1 gram of hydrocortisone into the cream base to achieve the desired concentration.

Ensuring Accuracy and Safety

Accuracy in calculations is paramount to patient safety. Always double-check your work and use reliable tools, such as calculators or pharmacy software, to verify your results. It's also important to stay up-to-date with guidelines and best practices, as these can change over time.

Practice Problems and Real-World Scenarios

To build confidence and proficiency in dosage calculations, practice regularly with real-world scenarios. Engage in exercises that cover a range of situations, from simple conversions to complex compounding tasks. Collaborate with colleagues to discuss challenging cases and share strategies for accurate calculations.

Detailed calculations for drug dosages are fundamental to the role of a pharmacy technician. Mastery of these skills ensures that patients receive the correct medication in the right amount, which is critical for effective treatment and patient safety. By understanding the underlying principles, practicing regularly, and maintaining meticulous attention to detail, you can excel in this essential aspect of pharmacy practice.

Advanced calculation scenarios in pharmacy often require more intricate mathematical approaches and a deeper understanding of pharmacokinetics and pharmacodynamics. These calculations are essential for tailoring drug regimens to individual patient needs, particularly in specialized fields such as oncology, pediatrics, and critical care. In this subchapter, we will explore complex scenarios that demand advanced calculation skills, providing real-world examples to illustrate these principles.

Pharmacokinetic Calculations

Pharmacokinetics involves the study of how a drug moves through the body, which includes absorption, distribution, metabolism, and excretion. Understanding these processes allows pharmacists to optimize dosing regimens for individual patients.

1. Calculating Clearance and Half-Life

Clearance (CL) is a measure of the body's ability to eliminate a drug, while the half-life ($t\frac{1}{2}$) is the time it takes for the plasma concentration of a drug to reduce by half. The formula for clearance is:

$$CL = \frac{Dose}{AUC}$$

where AUC is the area under the plasma concentration-time curve.

For half-life, the formula is:

$$t\frac{1}{2} = \frac{0.693 \times Vd}{CL}$$

where Vd is the volume of distribution.

Example:

A patient receives a 500 mg dose of a drug intravenously, and the AUC is found to be 50 mg·h/L. Calculate the clearance.

$$CL = \frac{500\,\text{mg}}{50\,\text{mg·h/L}} = 10\,\text{L/h}$$

If the volume of distribution (Vd) is 20 L, the half-life is:

$$t\frac{1}{2} = \frac{0.693 \times 20\,\text{L}}{10\,\text{L/h}} = 1.386\,\text{h}$$

2. Loading Dose and Maintenance Dose

The loading dose (LD) is used to quickly achieve the desired plasma concentration, while the maintenance dose (MD) maintains this concentration. The formula for the loading dose is:

$$LD = \frac{C_{desired} \times Vd}{F}$$

where $C_{desired}$ is the desired plasma concentration and F is the bioavailability.

The maintenance dose is calculated as:

$$MD = \frac{CL \times C_{desired} \times \tau}{F}$$

where τ is the dosing interval.

Example:

For a drug with a desired plasma concentration of 10 mg/L, a Vd of 40 L, and an oral bioavailability (F) of 0.8, the loading dose is:

$$LD = \frac{10 \text{ mg/L} \times 40 \text{ L}}{0.8} = 500 \text{ mg}$$

If the clearance is 5 L/h and the dosing interval is 12 hours:

$$MD = \frac{5 \text{ L/h} \times 10 \text{ mg/L} \times 12 \text{ h}}{0.8} = 750 \text{ mg}$$

Complex Intravenous (IV) Infusion Calculations

Intravenous infusions often require precise calculations to ensure the correct dosage over a specific time period, especially for drugs with narrow therapeutic windows.

Example: Continuous IV Infusion

A patient needs a continuous infusion of a medication at a rate of 5 mg/h. The solution is prepared with a concentration of 100 mg in 500 mL of IV fluid. Calculate the infusion rate in mL/h.

First, determine the concentration in mg/mL:

$$\text{Concentration} = \frac{100 \text{ mg}}{500 \text{ mL}} = 0.2 \text{ mg/mL}$$

Then, calculate the infusion rate:

$$\text{Infusion Rate} = \frac{5 \text{ mg/h}}{0.2 \text{ mg/mL}} = 25 \text{ mL/h}$$

Pediatric Dosing Adjustments

Pediatric dosing often requires adjustments based on weight, age, and surface area. These calculations ensure that children receive safe and effective doses tailored to their unique physiology.

Example: Body Surface Area (BSA) Dosing

For a pediatric patient with a BSA of 0.75 m², if the recommended dose of a medication is 150 mg/m², calculate the appropriate dose.

$$\text{Dose} = 0.75 \text{ m}^2 \times 150 \text{ mg/m}^2 = 112.5 \text{ mg}$$

Renal and Hepatic Dose Adjustments

Patients with renal or hepatic impairments often require dosage adjustments to prevent toxicity. These adjustments are based on the patient's creatinine clearance (CrCl) or liver function tests.

Example: Adjusting for Renal Impairment

A patient with a CrCl of 30 mL/min requires a drug that is normally dosed at 100 mg every 12 hours for patients with normal renal function (CrCl ≥ 80 mL/min). The dose needs to be adjusted according to renal function.

If the dosing adjustment guideline suggests reducing the dose to 50% for CrCl between 15-50 mL/min:

$$\text{Adjusted Dose} = 100 \text{ mg} \times 0.5 = 50 \text{ mg}$$

Thus, the new dosing regimen is 50 mg every 12 hours.

Compounding High-Risk Medications

Compounding high-risk medications, such as chemotherapy agents, requires precise calculations to ensure safety and efficacy.

Example: Chemotherapy Compounding

A patient requires a chemotherapy agent at a dose of 20 mg/m². The patient's BSA is 1.8 m², and the drug concentration is 10 mg/mL. Calculate the volume of the chemotherapy agent needed.

$$\text{Dose} = 20 \text{ mg/m}^2 \times 1.8 \text{ m}^2 = 36 \text{ mg}$$

$$\text{Volume} = \frac{36 \text{ mg}}{10 \text{ mg/mL}} = 3.6 \text{ mL}$$

Total Parenteral Nutrition (TPN) Calculations

TPN involves providing nutrition intravenously, which requires complex calculations to ensure the correct balance of nutrients.

Example: Calculating Macronutrient Requirements

For a patient receiving TPN, the required macronutrients are as follows: 1.5 g/kg/day of protein, 25 kcal/kg/day of carbohydrates, and 1 g/kg/day of fat. The patient weighs 70 kg.

Calculate the daily amounts of protein, carbohydrates, and fat:

$$\text{Protein} = 1.5 \text{ g/kg/day} \times 70 \text{ kg} = 105 \text{ g/day}$$

$$\text{Carbohydrates} = 25 \text{ kcal/kg/day} \times 70 \text{ kg} = 1750 \text{ kcal/day}$$

Assuming carbohydrates provide 4 kcal/g:

$$\text{Carbohydrates} = \frac{1750 \text{ kcal/day}}{4 \text{ kcal/g}} = 437.5 \text{ g/day}$$

$$\text{Fat} = 1 \text{ g/kg/day} \times 70 \text{ kg} = 70 \text{ g/day}$$

Ensuring Accuracy and Safety in Advanced Calculations

Accuracy is paramount in advanced pharmacy calculations. Always double-check your calculations and use reliable tools, such as calculators or pharmacy software, to verify your results. Collaborating with colleagues to review calculations can also help catch errors and ensure patient safety.

Advanced calculation scenarios in pharmacy require a deep understanding of mathematical principles and pharmacokinetics. These calculations are essential for tailoring drug regimens to individual patient needs, particularly in specialized fields such as oncology, pediatrics, and critical care. By mastering these advanced skills, pharmacy technicians can ensure precise dosing, optimize therapeutic outcomes, and enhance patient safety. Regular practice and continuous learning are key to maintaining proficiency in these complex calculations, ultimately contributing to the highest standards of patient care.

STEP-BY-STEP GUIDES TO MASTERING COMPOUNDING CALCULATIONS

Mastering compounding calculations is essential for any pharmacy technician involved in preparing customized medications. Whether you're adjusting dosages, mixing ingredients, or creating formulations from scratch, accurate calculations ensure patient safety and therapeutic efficacy. This subchapter provides a step-by-step guide to mastering the various aspects of compounding calculations, helping you gain confidence and precision in this critical area of pharmacy practice.

Understanding the Basics

Compounding involves creating pharmaceutical products tailored to specific patient needs. This often means working with different concentrations, volumes, and weights. The fundamental principle is ensuring that the final product contains the correct dosage of each ingredient.

Step 1: Converting Units

One of the first steps in compounding calculations is converting units. This is crucial because ingredients may come in different units than those needed for the final preparation.

For example, if a prescription requires 0.5 grams of a substance, but you have the substance in milligrams, you need to convert grams to milligrams:

$$0.5 \text{ grams} \times 1000 \text{ mg/gram} = 500 \text{ mg}$$

Similarly, if a prescription requires 100 mL of a solution, but you have the substance in liters, convert liters to milliliters:

$$1 \text{ liter} = 1000 \text{ mL}$$

Step 2: Calculating Percentages

Often, compounds are prepared as percentage solutions, where the concentration is expressed as a percentage of the total volume or weight. For instance, a 5% cream means there are 5 grams of active ingredient in 100 grams of the cream.

To calculate the amount of active ingredient in a specific volume:

$$\text{Amount of Active Ingredient} = \text{Percentage} \times \text{Total Volume or Weight}$$

For a 5% cream, if you need 200 grams of the cream:

Step 3: Using the Alligation Method

The alligation method is used for mixing solutions of different concentrations to achieve a desired concentration. This is particularly useful when you have two solutions and need to prepare a new solution with a specific intermediate concentration.

Example:

You have a 10% solution and a 2% solution, and you need to prepare 100 mL of a 5% solution.

1. Subtract the desired concentration from the higher concentration (10% - 5% = 5).
2. Subtract the lower concentration from the desired concentration (5% - 2% = 3).

These differences (5 and 3) indicate the ratio of the two solutions needed:

$$\text{Ratio} = 5 : 3$$

So, for 100 mL of a 5% solution, you need:

$$\frac{5}{5+3} \times 100 \text{ mL} = \frac{5}{8} \times 100 \text{ mL} = 62.5 \text{ mL}$$

$$\frac{3}{5+3} \times 100 \text{ mL} = \frac{3}{8} \times 100 \text{ mL} = 37.5 \text{ mL}$$

Step 4: Calculating Dosage for Compounded Medications

When compounding medications, it's essential to calculate the correct dosage for each ingredient. This often involves working with ratios and proportions.

Example:

You need to prepare 50 mL of a cough syrup containing 10 mg/mL of dextromethorphan. How much dextromethorphan is needed?

$$\text{Amount of Active Ingredient} = \text{Concentration} \times \text{Total Volume}$$

$$10 \text{ mg/mL} \times 50 \text{ mL} = 500 \text{ mg of dextromethorphan}$$

Step 5: Adjusting for Specific Patient Needs

Sometimes, you'll need to adjust formulations for specific patient needs, such as weight-based dosing for pediatric patients.

Example:

A pediatric patient weighing 20 kg needs a medication at a dose of 2 mg/kg/day, divided into two doses. You need to prepare a suspension.

1. Calculate the total daily dose:

$$2 \text{ mg/kg/day} \times 20 \text{ kg} = 40 \text{ mg/day}$$

2. Divide the total dose into two doses:

$$\frac{40 \text{ mg/day}}{2} = 20 \text{ mg/dose}$$

If the suspension concentration is 5 mg/mL:

$$\frac{20 \text{ mg}}{5 \text{ mg/mL}} = 4 \text{ mL per dose}$$

Step 6: Dilution and Concentration Adjustments

When compounding, you might need to dilute or concentrate a solution to achieve the desired strength.

Example:

You need to dilute a 10% solution to make 100 mL of a 1% solution.

1. Calculate the amount of the 10% solution needed:

$$C_1 \times V_1 = C_2 \times V_2$$
$$10\% \times V_1 = 1\% \times 100 \text{ mL}$$
$$V_1 = \frac{1 \times 100}{10} = 10 \text{ mL}$$

2. Add enough diluent to reach the final volume:

$$100 \text{ mL} - 10 \text{ mL} = 90 \text{ mL of diluent}$$

Step 7: Preparing Powders and Capsules

Compounding often involves preparing powders or capsules, which requires calculating the correct amount of each ingredient and ensuring uniform distribution.

Example:

You need to prepare 30 capsules, each containing 250 mg of an active ingredient.

1. Calculate the total amount needed:

$$250 \text{ mg/capsule} \times 30 \text{ capsules} = 7500 \text{ mg} = 7.5 \text{ g}$$

2. If the bulk powder has a density of 0.5 g/mL, calculate the volume needed:

$$\frac{7.5 \text{ g}}{0.5 \text{ g/mL}} = 15 \text{ mL}$$

Practical Tips for Accuracy

1. **Double-Check Calculations:** Always verify your calculations. A small mistake can lead to significant errors in the final product.
2. **Use Reliable Tools:** Utilize calculators, software, and references to ensure accuracy.
3. **Document Processes:** Keep detailed records of your calculations and compounding procedures.
4. **Stay Informed:** Continuously update your knowledge and skills through ongoing education and practice.

Mastering compounding calculations is a vital skill for pharmacy technicians, ensuring that patients receive safe and effective medications tailored to their needs. By following these step-by-step guides and practicing regularly, you can build confidence and precision in your compounding work. Accurate calculations not only enhance patient safety but also contribute to the overall quality of care provided by the pharmacy. Through diligent practice and attention to detail, you can excel in this essential aspect of pharmacy practice, ensuring that every compounded medication meets the highest standards of accuracy and efficacy.

STRATEGIES FOR EFFICIENTLY SOLVING PHARMACEUTICAL CONVERSIONS

Efficiently solving pharmaceutical conversions is a fundamental skill for pharmacy technicians. This ability ensures the correct preparation and dispensing of medications, which is crucial for patient safety and therapeutic efficacy. In this subchapter, we'll explore various strategies to master pharmaceutical conversions, focusing on practical methods and real-world examples.

Understanding the Basics

Pharmaceutical conversions involve changing one unit of measurement to another, such as converting milligrams to grams or milliliters to liters. A solid understanding of these conversions is essential for accurate medication dosing and preparation.

Step 1: Mastering Common Conversion Factors

Familiarity with common conversion factors is the first step toward efficient conversions. Some of the most frequently used conversion factors in pharmacy include:

- 1 gram (g) = 1000 milligrams (mg)
- 1 liter (L) = 1000 milliliters (mL)
- 1 kilogram (kg) = 1000 grams (g)
- 1 milliliter (mL) = 1 cubic centimeter (cc)

Having these conversions at your fingertips will streamline your calculations and reduce the risk of errors.

Step 2: Using Dimensional Analysis

Dimensional analysis, also known as the factor-label method, is a powerful tool for performing conversions. This method involves multiplying the quantity to be converted by one or more conversion factors arranged so that the units cancel out, leaving the desired unit.

Example:

Convert 500 milligrams to grams.

$$500 \text{ mg} \times \frac{1 \text{ g}}{1000 \text{ mg}} = 0.5 \text{ g}$$

In this example, the milligrams cancel out, and the result is in grams.

Step 3: Practicing With Real-World Scenarios

Applying conversion skills to real-world scenarios helps reinforce your understanding and improve your efficiency. Let's explore a few practical examples.

Converting Dosages

A prescription requires 0.75 grams of a medication. The available stock is in milligrams. Convert the required dose to milligrams.

$$0.75 \text{ g} \times 1000 \text{ mg/g} = 750 \text{ mg}$$

This conversion ensures you dispense the correct amount of medication.

Volume Conversions

You need to prepare a 250 mL solution, but your measuring tool is calibrated in liters. Convert the required volume to liters.

$$250 \text{ mL} \times \frac{1 \text{ L}}{1000 \text{ mL}} = 0.25 \text{ L}$$

By converting to liters, you can accurately measure the solution with the available tool.

Step 4: Utilizing Proportions

Proportions are another effective method for solving pharmaceutical conversions. This approach involves setting up two ratios and solving for the unknown quantity.

Example:

If 10 mL of a solution contains 50 mg of a drug, how much drug is in 25 mL of the solution?

Set up the proportion:

$$\frac{50 \text{ mg}}{10 \text{ mL}} = \frac{x \text{ mg}}{25 \text{ mL}}$$

Solve for x:

$$x = \frac{50 \text{ mg} \times 25 \text{ mL}}{10 \text{ mL}} = 125 \text{ mg}$$

Step 5: Converting Between Measurement Systems

Pharmacy technicians often need to convert between different measurement systems, such as metric to imperial units. Understanding these conversions is crucial for accurate medication preparation.

Common Conversions:

- 1 inch = 2.54 centimeters (cm)
- 1 ounce (oz) = 28.35 grams (g)
- 1 pound (lb) = 0.45 kilograms (kg)

Example:

Convert 5 ounces to grams.

$$5 \text{ oz} \times 28.35 \text{ g/oz} = 141.75 \text{ g}$$

Step 6: Converting Concentrations

Converting concentrations is essential when preparing solutions of different strengths. This involves understanding and applying percentage strength, ratio strength, and molarity.

Percentage Strength

Percentage strength is the amount of solute (active ingredient) in 100 parts of solution.

Example:

Convert a 10% solution to mg/mL.

A 10% solution means 10 grams of solute in 100 mL of solution.

$$10 \text{ g} \times \frac{1000 \text{ mg}}{1 \text{ g}} = 10,000 \text{ mg}$$

$$10,000 \text{ mg}/100 \text{ mL} = 100 \text{ mg/mL}$$

Ratio Strength

Ratio strength expresses the concentration as a ratio of solute to solvent.

Example:

Convert a 1:500 solution to mg/mL.

A 1:500 solution means 1 gram of solute in 500 mL of solution.

$$1 \text{ g} \times \frac{1000 \text{ mg}}{1 \text{ g}} = 1000 \text{ mg}$$

$$1000 \text{ mg}/500 \text{ mL} = 2 \text{ mg/mL}$$

Step 7: Converting Infusion Rates

Infusion rate conversions are critical for intravenous therapies, ensuring that medications are delivered at the correct rate.

Example:

Convert an infusion rate of 50 mL/hour to drops per minute (gtt/min) if the drop factor is 20 drops/mL.

$$50 \text{ mL/hour} \times \frac{20 \text{ gtt}}{1 \text{ mL}} = 1000 \text{ gtt/hour}$$

Convert to minutes:

$$1000 \text{ gtt/hour} \times \frac{1 \text{ hour}}{60 \text{ minutes}} \approx 16.67 \text{ gtt/min}$$

Practice and Application

To build proficiency in pharmaceutical conversions, practice regularly with a variety of scenarios. Here are some tips to help you master these skills:

1. **Use Real Prescriptions:** Practice conversions using actual prescriptions or case studies. This will help you understand the practical applications of these skills.
2. **Work in Groups:** Collaborate with colleagues to solve conversion problems. Discussing different approaches and techniques can enhance your understanding.
3. **Utilize Technology:** Take advantage of pharmacy software and apps that assist with conversions. These tools can provide quick, accurate results and help you double-check your calculations.
4. **Continual Learning:** Stay updated with the latest best practices and guidelines in pharmacy math. Regularly review and practice different types of conversions to keep your skills sharp.

Efficiently solving pharmaceutical conversions is an essential skill for pharmacy technicians. By mastering common conversion factors, using dimensional analysis, practicing with real-world scenarios, and applying various methods like proportions and unit conversions, you can ensure accuracy and safety in medication preparation and dispensing. Regular practice and a solid understanding of these techniques will enhance your proficiency and confidence in handling pharmaceutical calculations, ultimately contributing to the highest standards of patient care and safety.

PRACTICE EXERCISES WITH REAL-WORLD SCENARIOS

Practicing with real-world scenarios is an effective way to hone your pharmacy math skills and prepare for the challenges you'll face in the field. These exercises not only test your knowledge but also improve your problem-solving abilities and attention to detail. Let's explore various practice exercises based on real-world scenarios, designed to reinforce your understanding of pharmacy math basics.

Scenario 1: Dosage Calculation for a Pediatric Patient

A pediatric patient weighing 18 kg requires an antibiotic that is dosed at 25 mg/kg/day, divided into two doses.

1. Calculate the total daily dose.
2. Determine the dose per administration.

Solution:

1. **Total daily dose:**

$$25 \text{ mg/kg/day} \times 18 \text{ kg} = 450 \text{ mg/day}$$

2. **Dose per administration:**

$$\frac{450 \text{ mg/day}}{2} = 225 \text{ mg per dose}$$

Scenario 2: IV Infusion Rate

A patient needs to receive 1 gram of a medication over 4 hours. The medication is available in a concentration of 250 mg/50 mL. Calculate the infusion rate in mL/hour.

Solution:

1. **Convert grams to milligrams:**

   $$1 \text{ gram} = 1000 \text{ mg}$$

2. **Calculate the volume needed:**

   $$\frac{1000 \text{ mg}}{250 \text{ mg}} \times 50 \text{ mL} = 200 \text{ mL}$$

3. **Determine the infusion rate:**

   $$\frac{200 \text{ mL}}{4 \text{ hours}} = 50 \text{ mL/hour}$$

Scenario 3: Preparing a Solution

A prescription calls for 300 mL of a 5% dextrose solution. You have a stock solution of 25% dextrose. How much of the stock solution and how much diluent do you need?

Solution:

1. **Use the dilution formula:**

   $$C_1 \times V_1 = C_2 \times V_2$$

   $$25\% \times V_1 = 5\% \times 300 \text{ mL}$$

   $$V_1 = \frac{5 \times 300}{25} = 60 \text{ mL}$$

2. **Calculate the amount of diluent:**

   $$300 \text{ mL} - 60 \text{ mL} = 240 \text{ mL}$$

Scenario 4: Compounding a Cream

You need to prepare 100 grams of a 2% hydrocortisone cream. How much hydrocortisone and how much cream base do you need?

Solution:

1. **Calculate the amount of hydrocortisone:**

    $2\% \times 100 \text{ grams} = 2 \text{ grams}$

2. **Calculate the amount of cream base:**

    $100 \text{ grams} - 2 \text{ grams} = 98 \text{ grams}$

Scenario 5: Calculating Molarity

You need to prepare 500 mL of a 1 M NaCl solution. The molecular weight of NaCl is 58.44 g/mol. How much NaCl do you need?

Solution:

1. **Calculate the amount of NaCl needed:**

    $$\text{Molarity} \times \text{Volume (L)} \times \text{Molecular Weight (g/mol)}$$

    $1 \text{ M} \times 0.5 \text{ L} \times 58.44 \text{ g/mol} = 29.22 \text{ grams}$

Scenario 6: Adjusting a Dose for Renal Function

A patient with a creatinine clearance of 30 mL/min needs a drug dosed at 100 mg every 8 hours. The dose should be reduced by 50% for a creatinine clearance of 30 mL/min. Calculate the adjusted dose.

Solution:

1. **Calculate the adjusted dose:**

    $100 \text{ mg} \times 0.5 = 50 \text{ mg every 8 hours}$

Scenario 7: Converting Between Systems

Convert 5 milliliters to teaspoons, knowing that 1 teaspoon equals 5 milliliters.

Solution:

$$5 \text{ mL} \times \frac{1 \text{ teaspoon}}{5 \text{ mL}} = 1 \text{ teaspoon}$$

Scenario 8: Preparing a Suspension

A prescription calls for 150 mL of a 4 mg/mL suspension. You have 100 mg tablets available. How many tablets are needed to prepare the suspension?

Solution:

1. Calculate the total amount of active ingredient needed:

$$4 \text{ mg/mL} \times 150 \text{ mL} = 600 \text{ mg}$$

2. Calculate the number of tablets needed:

$$\frac{600 \text{ mg}}{100 \text{ mg/tablet}} = 6 \text{ tablets}$$

Scenario 9: Reconstituting a Powder

A vial contains 1 gram of a powdered drug. After reconstitution with 10 mL of diluent, what is the concentration of the solution?

Solution:

1. Calculate the concentration:

$$\frac{1000 \text{ mg}}{10 \text{ mL}} = 100 \text{ mg/mL}$$

Scenario 10: Mixing Two Solutions

You have 150 mL of a 20% solution and need to dilute it to a 10% solution. How much diluent should you add?

Solution:

1. Use the dilution formula:

$$C_1 \times V_1 = C_2 \times V_2$$

$$20\% \times 150 \text{ mL} = 10\% \times V_2$$

$$V_2 = \frac{20 \times 150}{10} = 300 \text{ mL}$$

2. Calculate the amount of diluent to add:

$$300 \text{ mL} - 150 \text{ mL} = 150 \text{ mL}$$

Practice Makes Perfect

Working through these scenarios will build your confidence and competence in performing pharmaceutical calculations. Regular practice helps solidify these concepts and ensures you're prepared for the varied and often complex tasks you'll encounter in a pharmacy setting.

Tips for Success

1. **Double-Check Your Work:** Always verify your calculations to avoid errors.
2. **Stay Organized:** Keep your work neat and organized to reduce mistakes.
3. **Use Reliable Tools:** Utilize calculators, conversion charts, and pharmacy software to assist with accuracy.
4. **Keep Learning:** Continuously update your knowledge and skills through practice and education.

Practice exercises based on real-world scenarios are invaluable for mastering pharmacy math basics. By applying these strategies and working through diverse problems, you enhance your ability to perform accurate calculations, ensuring the safe and effective preparation and dispensing of medications. Through consistent practice and a commitment to precision, you can excel in this crucial aspect of pharmacy practice, contributing to the highest standards of patient care and safety.

SOLVING COMMON MATHEMATICAL PROBLEMS IN PHARMACY

In pharmacy practice, encountering and solving mathematical problems is a routine part of ensuring accurate and safe medication dispensing. From dosage calculations to dilution and concentration adjustments, these mathematical skills are crucial. In this subchapter, we'll explore common mathematical problems in pharmacy and provide practical strategies to solve them effectively.

Dosage Calculations

One of the most frequent tasks in pharmacy is calculating the correct dosage of medication. This involves understanding the relationship between the dose, the concentration of the drug, and the volume required.

Example: Dosage for a Pediatric Patient

A pediatric patient weighing 15 kg requires a medication dosed at 10 mg/kg/day, divided into two doses.

1. **Calculate the total daily dose:**

$$10 \text{ mg/kg/day} \times 15 \text{ kg} = 150 \text{ mg/day}$$

2. **Calculate the dose per administration:**

$$\frac{150 \text{ mg}}{2} = 75 \text{ mg per dose}$$

Example: Dosage Based on Body Surface Area

A medication is dosed at 100 mg/m² for a patient with a body surface area (BSA) of 1.5 m².

1. **Calculate the total dose:**

$$100 \text{ mg/m}^2 \times 1.5 \text{ m}^2 = 150 \text{ mg}$$

Conversion Between Units

Pharmacy technicians often need to convert between different units of measurement, such as grams to milligrams or liters to milliliters. Understanding and quickly performing these conversions is essential.

Example: Converting Milligrams to Grams

Convert 500 mg to grams.

$$500 \text{ mg} \times \frac{1 \text{ g}}{1000 \text{ mg}} = 0.5 \text{ g}$$

Example: Converting Milliliters to Liters

Convert 250 mL to liters.

$$250 \text{ mL} \times \frac{1 \text{ L}}{1000 \text{ mL}} = 0.25 \text{ L}$$

Dilution and Concentration Adjustments

Adjusting the concentration of solutions is a common task, especially when preparing medications for specific patient needs. The key is to use the dilution formula correctly.

Example: Preparing a Diluted Solution

You need to prepare 100 mL of a 5% solution from a 20% stock solution.

1. **Calculate the amount of stock solution needed:**

$$C_1 \times V_1 = C_2 \times V_2$$
$$20\% \times V_1 = 5\% \times 100 \text{ mL}$$
$$V_1 = \frac{5 \times 100}{20} = 25 \text{ mL}$$

2. **Calculate the amount of diluent to add:**

$$100 \text{ mL} - 25 \text{ mL} = 75 \text{ mL}$$

Alligation Method for Mixing Solutions

The alligation method is useful when mixing solutions of different concentrations to achieve a desired final concentration.

Example: Mixing Two Alcohol Solutions

You have a 70% alcohol solution and a 30% alcohol solution. You need 500 mL of a 50% alcohol solution.

1. **Determine the ratio:**

$$\text{High Concentration} - \text{Desired Concentration} = 70\% - 50\% = 20$$
$$\text{Desired Concentration} - \text{Low Concentration} = 50\% - 30\% = 20$$

2. **The ratio is 20:20, which simplifies to 1:1.**

3. **Calculate the volumes needed:**

$$\text{Volume of 70\% solution} = \frac{1}{1+1} \times 500\,\text{mL} = 250\,\text{mL}$$
$$\text{Volume of 30\% solution} = \frac{1}{1+1} \times 500\,\text{mL} = 250\,\text{mL}$$

Reconstitution of Powders

Reconstituting powders into liquids involves calculating the correct volume of diluent to add to achieve the desired concentration.

Example: Reconstituting an Antibiotic

A vial contains 500 mg of a powdered antibiotic. After adding 10 mL of sterile water, the concentration is 50 mg/mL.

1. **Verify the concentration:**

$$\frac{500\,\text{mg}}{10\,\text{mL}} = 50\,\text{mg/mL}$$

IV Infusion Rate Calculations

Calculating the infusion rate for intravenous medications is critical to ensure that patients receive the correct dose over a specific period.

Example: Calculating Infusion Rate

A patient needs an IV infusion of 1 gram of medication over 8 hours. The medication is available in a concentration of 200 mg/50 mL.

1. **Convert the dose to milligrams:**

$$1\,\text{g} = 1000\,\text{mg}$$

2. **Calculate the total volume needed:**

$$\frac{1000\,\text{mg}}{200\,\text{mg/50 mL}} \times 50\,\text{mL} = 250\,\text{mL}$$

3. **Calculate the infusion rate:**

$$\frac{250\,\text{mL}}{8\,\text{hours}} = 31.25\,\text{mL/hour}$$

Calculating Doses for Different Routes of Administration

Different routes of administration may require different dosage forms and calculations, such as converting from oral to intravenous administration.

Example: Converting Oral to IV Dose

A patient is receiving 300 mg of a drug orally. The IV equivalent is 80% of the oral dose. Calculate the IV dose.

1. Calculate the IV dose:

$$300 \text{ mg} \times 0.8 = 240 \text{ mg}$$

Percentage and Ratio Strength Calculations

Understanding how to calculate percentage and ratio strengths is essential for preparing solutions and compounds.

Example: Calculating Percentage Strength

Prepare 100 mL of a 15% w/v solution of sodium chloride.

1. Calculate the weight of sodium chloride needed:

$$15\% \times 100 \text{ mL} = 15 \text{ g}$$

Example: Calculating Ratio Strength

Convert a 1:1000 solution to a percentage strength.

1. Calculate the percentage strength:

$$\frac{1 \text{ part}}{1000 \text{ parts}} \times 100 = 0.1\%$$

Tackling Complex Calculations

Complex calculations often involve multiple steps and conversions. Breaking these problems down into manageable parts can simplify the process.

Example: Preparing a Compound Medication

You need to prepare 50 grams of a 2% hydrocortisone cream using a 10% stock solution.

1. **Calculate the amount of stock solution needed:**

$$C_1 \times V_1 = C_2 \times V_2$$
$$10\% \times V_1 = 2\% \times 50 \text{ grams}$$
$$V_1 = \frac{2 \times 50}{10} = 10 \text{ grams}$$

2. **Calculate the amount of base needed:**

$$50 \text{ grams} - 10 \text{ grams} = 40 \text{ grams of cream base}$$

Practice and Consistency

Regular practice is key to mastering these common mathematical problems in pharmacy. Working through varied scenarios helps reinforce your understanding and improve your problem-solving skills.

Solving common mathematical problems in pharmacy requires a blend of knowledge, practice, and precision. By mastering dosage calculations, unit conversions, dilution and concentration adjustments, reconstitution of powders, IV infusion rates, and more, pharmacy technicians can ensure accurate and safe medication preparation and dispensing. Continuous practice and a methodical approach to these problems will enhance your proficiency and confidence, ultimately contributing to better patient care and safety.

9. BEYOND THE PTCB EXAM

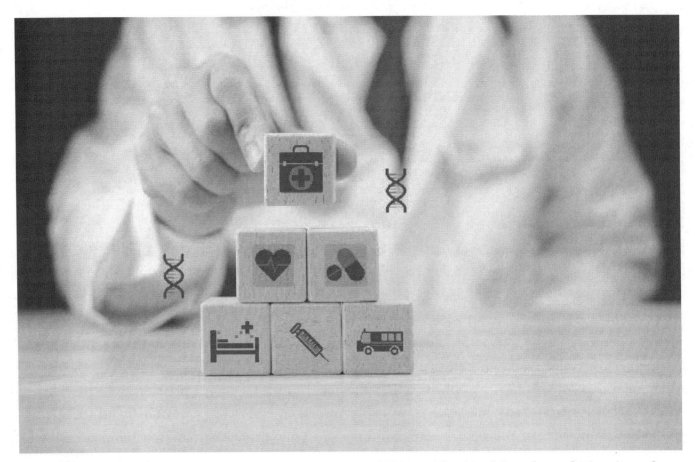

Congratulations! You've reached the final chapter of this guide, marking the culmination of your rigorous preparation for the PTCB exam. But passing the exam is just the beginning of your journey as a pharmacy technician. Beyond the PTCB exam lies a world of opportunities and challenges that will shape your career and professional growth.

Imagine standing at the threshold of your new career, equipped with knowledge and ready to make a meaningful impact on patients' lives. This chapter is designed to help you navigate the path ahead, offering insights into common study hurdles, opportunities for continuing education, and strategies for career advancement.

Embrace the possibilities that lie beyond certification. From pursuing specialized training and certifications to exploring diverse pharmacy settings, the choices you make will define your trajectory in this dynamic field. Whether you aim to deepen your expertise, take on leadership roles, or contribute to community health, the journey ahead promises growth and fulfillment. Let's explore the next steps in your professional adventure, ensuring you are well-prepared to excel and thrive in your career as a certified pharmacy technician.

ADDRESSING COMMON STUDY HURDLES

Studying for the PTCB exam is a significant undertaking, and many aspiring pharmacy technicians encounter various hurdles along the way. Addressing these common study challenges effectively can make a substantial difference in your preparation, ensuring you are well-equipped to pass the exam and succeed in your career. Let's explore some of these hurdles and practical strategies to overcome them, turning obstacles into opportunities for growth and learning.

Finding the Time to Study

One of the most common challenges is finding sufficient time to study amidst other responsibilities such as work, family, and personal commitments. Time management is crucial to balancing these demands and ensuring consistent study sessions.

Strategies for Effective Time Management:

1. **Create a Study Schedule:** Develop a realistic and flexible study plan that fits your daily routine. Allocate specific times for studying, and stick to this schedule as closely as possible. Break your study sessions into manageable chunks to avoid burnout.

2. **Prioritize Tasks:** Identify your most important tasks and focus on them first. Use tools like to-do lists or digital planners to keep track of your study goals and deadlines. Prioritizing tasks helps ensure you tackle the most critical subjects when you are most alert and focused.

3. **Utilize Short Breaks:** Make use of short breaks during your day to review flashcards or read through notes. Even a few minutes of focused study can be valuable and add up over time.

Dealing with Information Overload

The sheer volume of material covered in the PTCB exam can be overwhelming. From pharmacology to pharmacy law, it's easy to feel inundated with information.

Strategies to Manage Information Overload:

1. **Break It Down:** Divide the material into smaller, more manageable sections. Focus on one topic at a time, ensuring you thoroughly understand each before moving on. This approach makes the content less daunting and improves retention.

2. **Use Study Guides and Summaries:** Rely on concise study guides and summaries to distill the essential information. These resources provide a clear overview of key concepts and help you focus on the most important points.

3. **Active Learning Techniques:** Engage in active learning methods such as self-quizzing, teaching the material to someone else, or creating mind maps. These techniques enhance understanding and retention by involving multiple senses and cognitive processes.

Overcoming Procrastination

Procrastination is a common barrier to effective studying. It's easy to delay study sessions, especially when faced with challenging material or when feeling tired.

Strategies to Combat Procrastination:

1. **Set Specific Goals:** Establish clear, achievable goals for each study session. Having specific objectives gives you a sense of purpose and direction, making it easier to get started and stay focused.

2. **Create a Study Environment:** Designate a quiet, comfortable study area free from distractions. A consistent study space helps create a routine and signals to your brain that it's time to focus.

3. **Reward Yourself:** Set up a reward system to motivate yourself. After completing a study session or reaching a milestone, treat yourself to something you enjoy, whether it's a favorite snack, a short walk, or a break to watch a show.

Handling Exam Anxiety

Exam anxiety can hinder your ability to study effectively and perform well on the test. It's important to address this anxiety proactively to ensure you can approach the exam with confidence.

Strategies to Reduce Exam Anxiety:

1. **Practice Relaxation Techniques:** Incorporate relaxation exercises such as deep breathing, meditation, or progressive muscle relaxation into your routine. These techniques help calm your mind and reduce stress.

2. **Simulate Exam Conditions:** Practice taking full-length practice exams under timed conditions. Simulating the exam environment helps you become familiar with the format and timing, reducing anxiety on the actual test day.

3. **Focus on Preparation, Not Perfection:** Remember that thorough preparation is the best way to build confidence. Focus on doing your best rather than aiming for perfection. Accept that mistakes are part of the learning process and use them as opportunities to improve.

Building Confidence in Challenging Subjects

Certain subjects, such as pharmacy calculations or pharmacology, can be particularly challenging. Building confidence in these areas requires targeted strategies and consistent practice.

Strategies to Master Challenging Subjects:

1. **Seek Additional Resources:** Use supplementary materials such as online tutorials, instructional videos, and study groups. Different explanations and perspectives can help clarify difficult concepts.

2. **Practice Regularly:** Consistent practice is key to mastering challenging subjects. Dedicate extra time to these areas, and work through practice problems regularly to reinforce your understanding.

3. **Ask for Help:** Don't hesitate to seek assistance from instructors, mentors, or peers. Discussing difficult topics with others can provide new insights and make the material more accessible.

Maintaining Motivation

Staying motivated throughout your study journey is essential for sustained progress. It's natural for motivation to fluctuate, but there are ways to keep it high.

Strategies to Maintain Motivation:

1. **Visualize Success:** Keep your end goal in mind. Visualize yourself passing the PTCB exam and starting your career as a certified pharmacy technician. This positive imagery can boost your motivation and commitment.

2. **Set Milestones:** Break your study plan into smaller milestones and celebrate each achievement. Recognizing your progress helps maintain enthusiasm and provides a sense of accomplishment.

3. **Stay Connected:** Join study groups or online forums where you can share experiences and tips with fellow candidates. A supportive community can provide encouragement and keep you motivated.

Balancing Study with Self-Care

While it's important to dedicate time and effort to studying, it's equally crucial to maintain your well-being. Balancing study with self-care helps ensure you stay healthy and focused.

Strategies for Balancing Study and Self-Care:

1. **Prioritize Sleep:** Ensure you get adequate rest each night. Quality sleep improves memory, concentration, and overall well-being, making your study sessions more productive.

2. **Stay Active:** Incorporate physical activity into your routine. Regular exercise reduces stress, boosts energy levels, and enhances cognitive function.

3. **Take Breaks:** Schedule regular breaks during your study sessions to rest and recharge. Short breaks can improve focus and prevent burnout.

Reflecting on Progress

Regularly reflecting on your progress helps you stay on track and make necessary adjustments to your study plan. It also reinforces your achievements and boosts confidence.

Strategies for Reflecting on Progress:

1. **Keep a Study Journal:** Document your study sessions, noting what you covered, what you found challenging, and what you accomplished. Reviewing your journal helps you recognize patterns and track your improvement.

2. **Set Review Sessions:** Periodically review previous material to reinforce your knowledge and identify any areas that need more attention. Regular reviews help solidify information in your long-term memory.

3. **Adjust as Needed:** Be flexible with your study plan. If certain strategies aren't working, don't hesitate to try new approaches. Adjusting your plan based on your progress ensures continuous improvement.

Addressing common study hurdles effectively is key to a successful PTCB exam preparation. By managing your time, dealing with information overload, overcoming procrastination, handling exam anxiety, building confidence in challenging subjects, maintaining motivation, balancing study with self-care, and reflecting on your progress, you can navigate the study journey with confidence and achieve your goal of becoming a certified pharmacy technician. Each hurdle is an opportunity to develop resilience and enhance your skills, preparing you not only for the exam but for a rewarding career in pharmacy.

Continuing education is a vital component of a successful and fulfilling career in pharmacy. As a pharmacy technician, staying current with advancements in the field, enhancing your skills, and broadening your knowledge are essential for providing high-quality patient care and advancing your professional development. This subchapter explores various opportunities for continuing education in pharmacy, offering insights into how you can keep learning and growing in your career.

Importance of Continuing Education

The healthcare landscape is constantly evolving, with new medications, technologies, and regulatory changes emerging regularly. Continuing education ensures that pharmacy technicians remain knowledgeable about the latest developments, maintain their certification, and improve their competencies. This commitment to lifelong learning not only enhances your professional skills but also contributes to better patient outcomes and increased job satisfaction.

Formal Education Programs

Pursuing formal education programs is a structured way to advance your knowledge and skills. Many institutions offer specialized courses and degree programs designed for pharmacy technicians.

1. **Certificate Programs:** Numerous colleges and universities offer certificate programs in specialized areas such as sterile compounding, oncology pharmacy, and medication therapy management. These programs typically involve a series of courses focused on a specific area of practice, providing in-depth knowledge and practical skills.

2. **Associate's Degree in Pharmacy Technology:** An associate's degree program offers a comprehensive education in pharmacy practice, including coursework in pharmacology, pharmacy law, and patient care. This degree can enhance your qualifications and open up opportunities for advanced roles in the field.

3. **Bachelor's Degree in Health Sciences or Related Fields:** For those looking to further expand their education, a bachelor's degree in health sciences, public health, or a related field can provide a broader understanding of healthcare and open doors to leadership positions.

Professional Development Courses

In addition to formal education programs, numerous professional development courses are available to help pharmacy technicians stay current with industry trends and enhance their skills.

1. **Continuing Education (CE) Credits:** To maintain your certification, you'll need to complete a certain number of CE credits regularly. These courses cover a wide range of topics, from new drug therapies to patient safety practices. CE credits can be earned through online courses, seminars, workshops, and conferences.

2. **Workshops and Seminars:** Many professional organizations and institutions offer workshops and seminars on various aspects of pharmacy practice. These events provide hands-on training and the opportunity to learn from experts in the field.

3. **Online Learning Platforms:** Numerous online platforms offer courses and modules specifically designed for pharmacy technicians. Websites like Coursera, Udemy, and Khan

Academy provide access to courses on pharmacology, healthcare management, and more, allowing you to learn at your own pace.

Specialized Certifications

Obtaining specialized certifications can enhance your expertise and demonstrate your commitment to professional development. These certifications can make you a more competitive candidate for advanced positions and specialized roles.

1. **Certified Compounded Sterile Preparation Technician (CSPT):** This certification, offered by the Pharmacy Technician Certification Board (PTCB), focuses on sterile compounding practices. It demonstrates your expertise in preparing sterile medications, a critical skill in many healthcare settings.

2. **Certified Pharmacy Technician (CPhT) Advanced:** This advanced certification recognizes pharmacy technicians who have completed additional training and education in specialized areas such as medication therapy management or hazardous drug handling.

3. **Oncology Pharmacy Technician Certification:** This certification, offered by various organizations, focuses on the specialized knowledge and skills required for working in oncology pharmacy. It covers topics such as chemotherapy preparation, patient safety, and supportive care.

Attending Conferences and Networking Events

Attending professional conferences and networking events is an excellent way to stay informed about the latest developments in pharmacy and connect with peers and industry leaders.

1. **National Pharmacy Technician Association (NPTA) Annual Conference:** This conference offers educational sessions, hands-on workshops, and networking opportunities for pharmacy technicians. It's a great way to learn about new trends and technologies in the field.

2. **American Society of Health-System Pharmacists (ASHP) Midyear Clinical Meeting:** This meeting is one of the largest gatherings of pharmacy professionals, providing extensive educational programming and opportunities to network with colleagues from across the country.

3. **Local and Regional Events:** Many local and regional pharmacy organizations host events and meetings that offer educational sessions and networking opportunities. These events are a convenient way to stay connected with the local pharmacy community.

Engaging in Research and Publication

Participating in research and contributing to professional publications can enhance your understanding of pharmacy practice and establish you as an expert in the field.

1. **Conducting Research:** Engaging in research projects allows you to explore new areas of interest, contribute to the advancement of pharmacy practice, and develop critical thinking skills. Collaborate with pharmacists, healthcare providers, and academic institutions to conduct meaningful research.

2. **Publishing Articles:** Writing articles for professional journals, newsletters, and online platforms is a great way to share your knowledge and insights with the pharmacy community. It also helps you stay current with the latest research and trends in the field.

Mentorship and Peer Learning

Learning from experienced colleagues and sharing knowledge with peers can provide valuable insights and support your professional growth.

1. **Mentorship Programs:** Seek out mentorship programs within your organization or professional associations. A mentor can provide guidance, support, and valuable advice based on their experience in the field.

2. **Peer Learning Groups:** Join or form peer learning groups with fellow pharmacy technicians. These groups can provide a platform for discussing challenging cases, sharing best practices, and supporting each other's professional development.

Employer-Sponsored Training

Many employers offer training programs and educational opportunities to support the professional development of their staff. Take advantage of these resources to enhance your skills and advance your career.

1. **In-House Training Programs:** Participate in training sessions offered by your employer. These programs often cover important topics such as new drug therapies, safety protocols, and workflow optimization.

2. **Tuition Reimbursement:** Some employers provide tuition reimbursement for employees pursuing further education. Check with your HR department to see if you are eligible for this benefit.

Continuing education is essential for pharmacy technicians who wish to stay current, expand their skills, and advance their careers. Whether through formal education programs, professional development courses, specialized certifications, conferences, research, mentorship, or employer-sponsored training, numerous opportunities exist to enhance your knowledge and expertise. Embrace these opportunities to grow professionally, improve patient care, and contribute to the evolving field of pharmacy. Lifelong learning is a journey that not only benefits you as a professional but also the patients and communities you serve.

CAREER ADVANCEMENT POST-CERTIFICATION

Achieving PTCB certification is a significant milestone in your career as a pharmacy technician. It validates your knowledge and skills, opening the door to numerous opportunities for professional growth and advancement. However, certification is just the beginning. To fully realize your potential and advance your career, you need to explore various pathways and strategies that can elevate your professional standing. This subchapter delves into the opportunities and strategies for career advancement post-certification.

Expanding Your Role in the Pharmacy

Once certified, consider taking on more responsibilities within your current workplace. Expanding your role can demonstrate your capabilities and commitment to your career.

1. **Specialization:** Specialize in a particular area of pharmacy practice such as sterile compounding, oncology, or pediatrics. Specialization requires additional training and education but can significantly enhance your expertise and make you an invaluable asset to your team.

2. **Leadership Roles:** Take on leadership roles within your pharmacy. This could include becoming a lead technician, overseeing inventory management, or coordinating technician schedules. Leadership roles provide valuable experience and can be a stepping stone to further advancement.

3. **Training and Mentoring:** Offer to train new technicians or mentor peers. Sharing your knowledge and experience not only helps others but also reinforces your own understanding and establishes you as a leader in your workplace.

Pursuing Additional Certifications

Earning additional certifications can enhance your qualifications and open up new career opportunities. Specialized certifications validate your skills in specific areas of pharmacy practice.

1. **Certified Compounded Sterile Preparation Technician (CSPT):** This certification focuses on sterile compounding, a critical area in many healthcare settings. It demonstrates your expertise in preparing sterile medications, enhancing your credentials and job prospects.

2. **Certified Pharmacy Technician (CPhT) Advanced:** An advanced certification recognizes additional training and expertise in specialized areas such as medication therapy management or hazardous drug handling. This can make you a more competitive candidate for advanced roles.

3. **Other Specialty Certifications:** Consider certifications in areas such as chemotherapy, immunization, or pharmacy informatics. Each certification enhances your skill set and broadens your career options.

Continuing Education and Formal Degrees

Continuing your education through formal degree programs can provide a deeper understanding of pharmacy and healthcare, opening up higher-level positions and career paths.

1. **Associate's Degree in Pharmacy Technology:** An associate's degree offers comprehensive training in pharmacy practice, including coursework in pharmacology, pharmacy law, and patient care. This degree can enhance your qualifications and prepare you for advanced roles.

2. **Bachelor's Degree in Health Sciences or Related Fields:** A bachelor's degree provides a broader understanding of healthcare and can lead to leadership positions or specialized roles within the pharmacy field.

3. **Advanced Degrees:** Pursuing a master's degree in healthcare administration, public health, or a related field can open doors to executive positions and other high-level roles within healthcare organizations.

Exploring Diverse Pharmacy Settings

Pharmacy technicians are needed in various settings beyond traditional retail pharmacies. Exploring different work environments can lead to exciting and fulfilling career opportunities.

1. **Hospital Pharmacies:** Working in a hospital pharmacy involves preparing and dispensing medications for inpatients, managing IV admixtures, and collaborating with healthcare teams. This setting offers a dynamic and fast-paced environment with opportunities for specialization.

2. **Long-Term Care Facilities:** Technicians in long-term care facilities manage medications for residents, ensuring they receive the correct dosages and addressing any medication-related issues. This role often involves close interaction with patients and healthcare providers.

3. **Compounding Pharmacies:** Specializing in compounding allows you to create customized medications tailored to individual patient needs. This setting requires precision and specialized knowledge, making it a rewarding area for advancement.

4. **Pharmacy Benefit Management (PBM) Companies:** Working for a PBM involves managing prescription drug benefits for insurance companies, processing claims, and ensuring compliance with regulations. This role offers a different perspective on pharmacy practice and can involve administrative and analytical skills.

Networking and Professional Associations

Networking is crucial for career advancement. Building connections with other professionals in the field can provide support, mentorship, and opportunities for growth.

1. **Join Professional Associations:** Associations such as the National Pharmacy Technician Association (NPTA) and the American Society of Health-System Pharmacists (ASHP) offer networking opportunities, educational resources, and professional development programs.

2. **Attend Conferences and Workshops:** Participate in conferences, workshops, and seminars to stay updated on industry trends, learn from experts, and connect with peers. These events can also provide opportunities to showcase your skills and knowledge.

3. **Engage in Online Communities:** Join online forums and social media groups related to pharmacy practice. Engaging in discussions, sharing insights, and seeking advice from other professionals can help you stay connected and informed.

Pursuing Management and Administrative Roles

Management and administrative roles offer the chance to influence the operations and direction of pharmacy practice. These positions often require additional skills in leadership, management, and communication.

1. **Pharmacy Manager:** As a pharmacy manager, you oversee the daily operations of the pharmacy, manage staff, handle budgets, and ensure compliance with regulations. This role requires strong leadership and organizational skills.

2. **Health Services Manager:** This position involves overseeing the delivery of healthcare services, managing budgets, and ensuring that the pharmacy complies with healthcare laws and regulations. A background in health services management or a related field can be beneficial.

3. **Compliance Officer:** Compliance officers ensure that the pharmacy adheres to all relevant laws and regulations. This role involves auditing practices, developing compliance programs, and training staff on regulatory requirements.

Embracing Technology and Innovation

The pharmacy field is continually evolving with advancements in technology and innovation. Embracing these changes can enhance your career prospects and allow you to contribute to the modernization of pharmacy practice.

1. **Pharmacy Informatics:** This specialty involves managing and utilizing health information systems to improve patient care and pharmacy operations. Technicians in this field work with electronic health records, medication management systems, and data analytics.

2. **Telepharmacy:** Telepharmacy allows for the provision of pharmacy services remotely, using telecommunications technology. This growing area offers new opportunities for providing care to underserved populations and improving access to pharmacy services.

3. **Automation and Robotics:** Automation in pharmacies can streamline processes, reduce errors, and improve efficiency. Technicians who are skilled in operating and managing automated systems are valuable assets to any pharmacy.

Developing Soft Skills

In addition to technical skills, developing soft skills such as communication, teamwork, and problem-solving is crucial for career advancement. These skills enhance your ability to interact with colleagues, patients, and other healthcare professionals effectively.

1. **Communication:** Effective communication is essential for providing excellent patient care and collaborating with healthcare teams. Focus on improving your verbal and written communication skills.

2. **Teamwork:** Working well with others is critical in a pharmacy setting. Develop your ability to collaborate, support your colleagues, and contribute to a positive work environment.

3. **Problem-Solving:** Strong problem-solving skills enable you to address challenges and find effective solutions. This skill is valuable in all aspects of pharmacy practice, from managing inventory to resolving patient issues.

Advancing your career post-certification involves a combination of expanding your role, pursuing additional certifications and education, exploring diverse pharmacy settings, networking, embracing technology, and developing soft skills. By taking proactive steps to enhance your knowledge, skills, and professional connections, you can achieve greater success and fulfillment in your career as a pharmacy technician. Your commitment to continuous learning and growth not only benefits you but also contributes to the overall improvement of patient care and the pharmacy profession.

SCAN THE QR CODE TO DOWNLOAD YOUR PRACTICE TESTS AND FLASHCARDS:

Made in the USA
Columbia, SC
08 November 2024

46031979R00072